Understanding Mental Health of Adolescent Girls

Nancy

TABLE OF CONTENTS

Title page

Bonafide Certificate

Declaration

Acknowledgement

Table of Contents

List of Tables

List of Figures

Abbreviations

Chapter No.	Title	Page No.
I	**Introduction**	**1-28**
II	**Review of Literature**	**29-67**
III	**Research Methodology**	**68-84**
IV	**Analysis and Interpretation**	**85-170**
V	**Findings, Suggestions and Conclusion**	**171-191**
	Bibliography	**192-211**
	Appendices	

List of Tables

LIST OF TABLES

Table No.	Title	Page No.
1	Table Depicting the Samples	78
2	Table Presenting Reliability Co-efficient.	79
3	Distribution of Respondents by their Personal Details	85
4	Table Demonstrating the Mental Health of the Respondents	90
5	Table Showing Respondents by their Home Environment	92
6	Table Indicating the Personality Traits of the Adolescent Girls	94
7	Anova Showing Mental Health and Medium of Instruction	96
8	Anova Presenting Age and Mental Health	97
9	Anova Indicating Mental health and Birth order	98
10	Anova Depicting Mental health and Father's Education	99
11	Anova Showing Mental health and Mother's Education	100
12	Anova Revealing Mental health and Family Monthly Income	101
13	Anova for Mental health and Total Number of Members in the Family	102
14	Table Showing the Feeling of Respondents on lack of confidence	103
15	Table Revealing the Feeling of Respondents on Getting Excited Easily	104
16	Classification showing the Inability of Respondents on Taking Quick Decisions	105
17	Table Presenting the Belief of Respondents that situations are Continuously Going against them	106
18	Table Showing the Affection and Attachment of the Respondents with their Neighbours	107
19	Table Demonstrating Respondents' opinion on Adjusting themselves as per Circumstances	108
20	Table Revealing the belief of the Respondents on losing Self respect	109
21	Classification of Respondents on Worrying About Trivial Matters	110

Table No.	Title	
22	Classification on feeling of hesitation of the Respondents in meeting others	111
23	Table Showing the feeling of the Respondents on doing duty well in adverse circumstances	112
24	Table Indicating the feeling of the Respondents on not able to fully utilize their ability in performing Duties	113
25	Table Presenting the feeling of the Respondents that even in adverse circumstances, they act without keeping in view of the real facts	114
26	Table Depicting the feeling of the Respondents on getting irritated	115
27	Table Revealing the opinion of the Respondents on feeling insecure	116
28	Table Showing the opinion of the Respondents on feeling worried about responsibilities	117
29	Table Demonstrating the opinion of Respondents on feeling depressed or dejected	118
30	Table Exhibiting the opinion of Respondents on utilizing reasoning in difficult times	120
31	Table Depicting the feeling of Respondents on keeping satisfactory relations with others	121
32	Table Presenting the feeling of inferiority complex of the Respondents	122
33	Classification Indicating the feeling of to be lost in the world of imagination by the Respondents	123
34	Table Exhibiting the anxiety of the Respondents about their future	124
35	Table Demonstrating the opinion of Respondents on getting enraged by the slightest unfavourable task	125
36	Table Presenting belief of the Respondents on their confidence level variation	126
37	Table Indicating the willingness of the Respondents to face and fight the problems of life	127
38	Table Depicting the belief of the Respondents on solving the problems by their self	128
39	Table Revealing the belief of the Respondents on being perplexed by their contradictory thoughts	129

Table No.	Title	Page No.
40	Table Exhibiting the opinion of the Respondents on not able to continue any task for long	130
41	Table Presenting the feeling of being secured admist of friends or groups by the Respondents	131
42	Table Demonstrating the opinion of the Respondents on the feeling that they not become hopeless	132
43	Classification Indicating the opinion of the Respondents on not getting influenced even by reasonable arguments	133
44	Table Revealing the feeling of the Respondents on being afraid of imaginary calamities	134
45	Table Exhibiting the feeling of the Respondents on whether world is a good place for living	135
46	Table Depicting the Respondents feeling on being fully enthusiastic on thinking about achieving self objectives	136
47	Distribution Showing the feeling of Respondents on do not getting disappointed with common worries of daily life	137
48	Table Demonstrating the feeling of respondents on their Mood Changes	138
49	Table Presenting the feeling of Respondents that their intimacy with their group community is increasing	139
50	Table Indicating the opinion of Respondents on feeling pleasure in taking responsibilities	140
51	Correlation Table for Mental health and Home environment of the Adolescent Girls	141
52	Correlation Table Presenting the Home environment and Personality Traits of the Adolescent Girls	142
53	Correlation Table Depicting Personality Traits and Mental health of the Respondents	143
54	Chi-Square Test Showing Home environment and Mental health of the Respondents	144
55	Chi-Square Test Demonstrating Personality traits and Mental health of Adolescent girls	146
56	T-Test Presenting Mental Health and Psychotism	148
57	T-Test Exhibiting Mental Health And Depression	149

Table No.	Title	Page No.
58	T-Test Representing Mental Health and Extroversion	150
59	T-Test Indicating Mental health and Emotional instability	151
60	T-Test Showing Mental Health and Social Desirability	152
61	Chi-Square Test Presenting Medium of Instruction and Total Members in Family	153
62	Chi-Square Test Displaying Medium of Instruction and Father's Education	154
63	Chi-Square Test Exhibiting Medium of Instruction and Mother's Education	155
64	Anova Test for Medium of instruction and Home environment	156
65	Anova Test Exhibiting Home environment and Age	157
66	Anova Test Showing Home environment and Birth Order	158
67	Anova Test Presenting Home environment and Father's Education	159
68	Anova Test Displaying Home environment and Mother's Education	160
69	Anova Test Demonstrating Home environment and Family Monthly Income	161
70	Anova Test Exhibiting Home environment and number of family members	162
71	Factor Analysis for home environment	163
72	Comparison Table Showing Mental Health score based on Personality dimension -Pychotism and home environment of the Respondents	166
73	Comparison table for Mental Health score based on Personality Dimension- Depression and home environment of the respondents	167
74	Comparison table Indicating Mental Health score based on Personality Dimension -Extroversion and home environment of the Respondents	168
75	Comparison table Presenting Mental Health score based on Personality Dimension - Emotional Instability and home environment of the Respondents	169
76	Comparison table for Mental Health score based on Personality Dimension - Social Desirability and home environment of the respondents	170

List of Figures

LIST OF FIGURES

Figure No.	Title	Page No.
1	Figure on Aspects Affecting Mental health of Children and Adolescents	27
2	Distribution of Respondents by their Age	87
3	Distribution of Respondents by their Birth order	88
4	Distribution of Respondents by their Family Monthly Income	89
5	Distribution of Respondents by their Mental Health	91
6	Distribution of Respondents by their Home Environment condition	93
7	Classification of Respondents by the personality Scores of the Adolescent girls	95
8	Distribution of Respondents on feeling Depressed or Dejected	119
9	Figure showing changes in Adolescent Girls	180
10	Figure Presenting Social work at a Glance	185
11	Figure Exhibiting Stress Relief Activities	190

Abbreviations

ABBREVIATIONS

ACE	-	Active/effective Contact with the Environment
ADHD	-	Attention deficit hyperactivity disorder
et al.	-	and others
etc	-	Et cetera
for e.g.	-	for example
i.e.	-	That is
IASSW	-	International Association of Schools of Social Work
IFSW	-	International Federation of Social Workers
LOC	-	Locus of Control
MH	-	Mental Health
MHC-SF	-	Mental Health Continuum – Short Form
PSS	-	Psycho Social Success
WHO	-	World health organization

CHAPTER 1

INTRODUCTION

Introduction

Well-being is a positive outcome that is meaningful for people and for many sectors of society, because it tells us that people perceive that, their lives are going on well. Good living conditions like food, housing, employment are fundamental to well-being. Tracking these conditions is important for public policy. However, many indicators that measure, living conditions fail to measure what people think and feel about their lives, such as the quality of their relationships, their positive emotions and resilience, the realization of their potential, or their overall satisfaction with life i.e., their 'well-being.' Well-being generally includes global judgments of life satisfaction and feelings ranging from depression to joy.

Relevance of Research in Social Work

Social work is a practice profession. As such, the major objective of social work research is to search for answers to questions raised regarding interventions or practice effectiveness. In other words, social work research attempts to provide knowledge about what interventions or treatments really help or hinder in the attaining social work goals. In addition, it also helps in searching for answers to problems or difficulties faced by social work practitioners in the practice of their profession. Ultimately it helps building knowledge base on social work theory and practice. Social work research also deals with problems faced by professional social workers, social work agencies and community in its concern with social work functions. It is obvious that in social work research, the study of a problem is from the point of view of social work and that of professional social work. The designing of research problems, data collection and its interpretation will have to be attempted in a manner that would be useful to professional social work which would add new knowledge to the social work theory and practice and improve the efficiency of professional social workers.

Mental Health

Mental health includes our emotional, psychological, and social well-being. It affects how we think, feel, and act. It also help to determine how we handle stress, relate to others, and make choices. Mental health is important at every stage of life, from childhood and adolescence through adulthood.

WHO (2001) defines mental health as a state of well-being in which the individual realizes his or her own abilities, cope with normal stresses of life, can work productively and fruitful and is able to make a contribution to his or her community.

Komrad (2012) asserts that "mental health problems affect all segments of society, regardless of age, gender, education, or ethnicity". Indeed, everyone experiences problems, and those problems can make us feel awful. They can negatively affect our thoughts, our emotions, and our behaviors. However, no matter the nature of bad times, mental health can be improved. Everyone has a fluctuating state of mental health. It's possible for someone living with mental illness to achieve a high degree of mental health. Likewise, it's possible for someone who does not have a mental illness to experience poor mental health.

Shah (1982) has stated that mental health is the most essential and inseparable component of health.

Soddy (1961) defines mental health as the internal balance of the individual, quality of relationship between individuals and the groups and between groups themselves.

Sigmund Freud (1880) gave a minimum, but a significal definition that a person is said to be mentally healthy if he could love and work.

According to Schriber (1951) mental health means the ability of the individual to pursue reasonable, purposeful goals, use his capacities and talents fruitfully such an individual experiences a sense of security, belongingness, being respected and has the knowledge that he is liked or loved, has a sense of self-respect and self-reliance. In addition he has learnt to respect others, to accept others, to live fairly and in peace with others.

Criterias of Mental Health

Criteria of mental health are:-

- Adequate contact with reality
- Control of thought and imagination

- Efficiency in work and play
- Social acceptance
- Positive self-concept
- A healthy emotional life.

An example of wellness model includes one developed by Myers, Sweeney, and Witner. It includes life tasks:-

- Essence or spirituality
- Work and leisure
- Love
- Self-direction – and twelve

Sub tasks:

- Sense of worth
- Sense of control
- Realistic beliefs
- Emotional awareness and coping
- Problem solving and creativity
- Sense of humour
- Nutrition
- Exercise
- Self-care
- Stress management
- Culture identity is identified as one of the characteristics of healthy functioning and a major component of wellness. The components provide a means of responding to the circumstances of life in a manner that promotes healthy functioning.

Theories on Mental Health

All the views on mental health is centered totally around the individual. It assumes that locus of functioning is situated within the individual and is independent of the environment.

Cognitive Revolution Theory

This theory assumes that the way in which people process information about environment is an important determinant of their mental health

Dual Factor Theory

Verma (1988) postulates that there are different set of factors that contributes to negative and positive mental health. Similarly, some factors when present contribute only to positive mental health but their absence does not necessarily mean a negative mental health. Positive mental health could be manifested as general feeling of well-being, self-confidence, personal competence, security, adjustment, originality, satisfaction etc. Positive mental health is not a mere sum total of all these desirable characters, but how these factors are organized to depict a person as a distinct entity from others, yet part of the society. So, mental health can be summed up as how people think, feel and act as they face life situations. It shows how people handle them and relate to one another.

Mental Health Status

Mental health status refers to the degrees of mental health that a person possesses. In order to measure mental health status of a person the following 15 points have to be taken into consideration.

Optimism

It is a tendency to look on the bright side of things and to anticipate the most favorable result. This can be measured by assessing the expectation about future and attitude towards pleasurable experiences.

Adaptability

It is flexibility in meeting changed circumstances or demands. It can be measured by testing whether the individual could get adjusted to various situations.

Sense of security

It is a feeling of having maintenance of condition necessary to need gratification. It indicates how far the individual has the feeling of sense of security.

Regularity of Habits

This approximately indicates how far the individual is regular in habits.

Perception of Reality

This is the process of getting to know the object in the environment. This can be tested by checking the individual's judgment about other's criticism, whether he is day dreaming etc.

Emotional Maturity

It is the degree to which an individual manifests behaviour appropriate to his age and intelligence level. This is assessed in terms of individual's behaviour in various situations (whether appropriate or not etc).

Social conformity

This is measured by assessing how far the individual is able to confirm or adjust to the norms and customs of the society

Freedom from sociopathic tendencies

Sociopathic tendencies are characterized by lack of social responsibility and inability to confirm to prevailing social norms even when such norms are adoptive.

Recreational pursuits

This indicates how far the individual engages in recreational activities.

Environmental Mastery

This variable approximately indicates the individual's ability to master his environment.

Positive attitude towards self

It is the attitude of having a good outlook for everything not only in other people but also everything he does.

Freedom from negativism

It consists of individual's ability to avoid the negative things related to one thing.

Freedom from Nervousness

This can be measured by assessing how for the individual is free from the state of emotional tension, restlessness and hypersensitivity.

Freedom from withdrawing tendencies

This is assessed by checking how far the individual is free from tendency for intellectual, emotional or physical deficits.

Concept of degree of freedom

This indicates approximately the individual concept of freedom

Early Warning Signs

Experiencing one or more of the following feelings or behaviors can be an early warning sign of a mental health problem:

- Eating or sleeping too much or too little
- Pulling away from people and usual activities
- Having low or no energy
- Feeling numb or like nothing matters
- Having unexplained aches and pains
- Feeling helpless or hopeless
- Smoking, drinking, or using drugs more than usual
- Feeling unusually confused, forgetful, on edge, angry, upset, worried, or scared
- Yelling or fighting with family and friends
- Experiencing severe mood swings that cause problems in relationships
- Having persistent thoughts and memories you can't get out of your head
- Hearing voices or believing things that are not true

- Thinking of harming yourself or others
- Inability to perform daily tasks like taking care of your kids or getting to work or school

Mental well-being

Mental health can be seen as an unstable continuum, where an individual's mental health may have many different possible values. Mental wellness is generally viewed as a positive attribute, even if the person does not have any diagnosed mental health condition. This definition of mental health highlights emotional well-being, the capacity to live a full and creative life, and the flexibility to deal with life's inevitable challenges. Some discussions are formulated in terms of contentment or happiness. Many therapeutic systems and self-help books offer methods and philosophies espousing strategies and techniques vaunted as effective for further improving the mental wellness. Positive psychology is increasingly prominent in mental health.

A holistic model of mental health generally includes concepts, based upon anthropological, psychological, religious and sociological perspectives, as well as theoretical perspectives from personality social, clinical, health and developmental psychology.

The tripartite model of mental well-being views mental well-being as encompassing three components of emotional well-being, social well-being, and psychological well-being. Emotional well-being is defined as having high levels of positive emotions, whereas social and psychological well-being are defined as the presence of psychological and social skills and abilities that contribute to optimal functioning in daily life. The model has received empirical support across cultures. The Mental Health Continuum-Short Form (MHC-SF) is the most widely used scale to measure the tripartite model of mental well-being.

Mental Illness

Mental illness is a health problem that significantly affects how a person thinks, behaves and interacts with other people. It is diagnosed according to standardized criteria.

A mental health problem also affects how a person thinks, feels, and behaves, but to a lesser extent than a mental illness.

Mental illnesses are of different types and degrees of severity. Some of the major types are:

- anxiety
- schizophrenia
- bipolar mood disorder
- personality disorders
- eating disorders
- depression

These illnesses may also be referred to as a mental disorder, mental impairment or psychiatric disability.

Causes of Mental Illness

Mental illness results from complex interactions between the mind, body and environment. Factors which can contribute to mental illness are:

- long-term and acute stress
- biological factors such as genetics, chemistry and hormones
- use of alcohol, drugs and other substances
- cognitive patterns such as constant negative thoughts and low self esteem
- social factors such as isolation, financial problems, family breakdown or violence

These factors can be minimized by a strong and supportive community environment.

Prevention

Mental health is conventionally defined as a hybrid of absence of a mental disorder and presence of well-being. Focus is increasing on preventing mental disorders. Prevention is beginning to appear in mental health strategies, including the 2004 WHO report "Prevention of Mental Disorders", the 2008 EU "Pact for Mental Health" and the 2011 US "National Prevention Strategy". Prevention of a disorder at a young age may significantly decrease the chances that a child will suffer from a disorder later in life, and shall be the most efficient and effective measure from a public health perspective. Prevention may require the regular consultation of a physician for at least twice a year to detect any signs that reveal any mental health concerns.

Children and young adults

Mental health and stability is a very important factor in a person's everyday life. Social skills, behavioural skills, and someone's way of thinking are just some of the things that the human brain develops at an early age. Learning how to interact with others and how to focus on certain subjects are essential lessons to learn from the time we can talk all the way to when we are so old that we can barely walk. However, there are some people out there who have difficulty with these kind of skills and behaving like an average person. This is a most likely the cause of having a mental illness. A mental illness is a wide range of conditions that affect a person's mood, thinking, and behavior.

The most common mental illnesses in children include, but are not limited to, ADHD, autism and anxiety disorder, as well as depression in older children and teens. Having a mental illness at a younger age is much different from having one in your thirties. Children's brains are still developing and will continue to develop until around the age of twenty-five. When a mental illness is thrown into the mix, it becomes significantly harder for a child to acquire the necessary skills and habits that people use throughout the day. For example, behavioral skills don't develop as fast as motor or sensory skills do. So when a child has an anxiety disorder, they begin to lack proper social interaction and associate many ordinary things with intense fear. This can be scary for the child because they don't necessarily understand why they act and think the way that they do. Many researchers say that parents should keep an eye on their child if they have any reason to believe that something is slightly off. If the children are evaluated earlier, they become more acquainted to their disorder and treating it becomes part of their daily routine. This is opposed to adults who might not recover as quickly because it is more difficult for them to adapt.

Mental illness affects not only the person themselves, but the people around them. Friends and family also play an important role in the child's mental health stability and treatment. If the child is young, parents are the ones who evaluate their child and decide whether or not they need some form of help. Friends are a support system for the child and family as a whole. Living with a mental disorder is never easy, so it's always important to have people around to make the days a little easier. However, there are negative factors that come with the social aspect of mental illness as well. Parents are sometimes held responsible for their child's own illness. People also say that the parents raised their children in a certain way or they acquired their behavior from them. Family and friends are sometimes so ashamed of the idea of being close to someone with a disorder that the child feels isolated and thinks that they have to hide their illness from others. When in reality, hiding it from people prevents the child from getting the right amount of social interaction and treatment in order to thrive in today's society.

Stigma is also a well-known factor in mental illness. Stigma is defined as "a mark of disgrace associated with a particular circumstance, quality, or person." Stigma is used especially when it comes to the mentally disabled. People have this assumption that everyone with a mental problem, no matter how mild or severe, is automatically considered destructive or a criminal person. Thanks to the media, this idea has been planted in our brains from a young age. Watching movies about teens with depression or children with Autism makes us think that all of the people that have a mental illness are like the ones on TV. In reality, the media displays an exaggerated version of most illnesses. Unfortunately, not many people know that, so they continue to belittle those with disorders. In a recent study, a majority of young people associate mental illness with extreme sadness or violence. Now that children are becoming more and more open to technology and the media itself, future generations will then continue to pair mental illness with negative thoughts. The media should be explaining that many people with disorders like ADHD and anxiety, with the right treatment, can live ordinary lives and should not be punished for something they cannot help.

Mental Health and Wellness

Positive mental health allows people to:

- Realize their full potential
- Cope with the stresses of life

- Work productively
- Make meaningful contributions to their communities

Ways to maintain positive mental health include:

- Getting professional help if you need it
- Connecting with others
- Staying positive
- Getting physically active
- Helping others
- Getting enough sleep
- Developing coping skills

Adolescence

Adolescence is a developmental transition between childhood and adulthood. It is the period from puberty until full adult status has been attained. There are also varying views on the actual time line of adolescence-especially about when it ends. Typically, we view adolescence beginning at puberty and ending at 18 or 21 years. Others suggest that there is a period of late adolescence that extends well into what is now known as the period of young adulthood.

Theories on Adolescence

G. Stanley Hall's Biogenetic Psychology of Adolescence

G. Stanley Hall (1844-1924), was the first psychologist to advance a psychology of adolescence in its own right and to use scientific methods to study them. He defined this period to begin at puberty at about 12 or 13 years, and end late, between 22 years to 25 years of age. Hall also described adolescence as a period of **Sturm und Drang," Storm and Stress."** In German literature, the period of Sturm und Drang includes the works of Schiller and the early writings of Goethe. It is a literary movement full of idealism, commitment to a goal, and revolution against the old, expression of personal feelings, passion and suffering. Hall saw an analogy between the objectives of this group of young writers at the turn of the eighteenth century and the psychological characteristics of adolescence.

According to Hall's analogy and expansion of Darwin's concept of biological "evolution." into a psychological theory of recapitulation, adolescence corresponds to a time when the human race was in a turbulent transitional stage. (Muuss, 1975, pp.33-35) In this theory, Hall stated that the experiential history of the human species had become part of the genetic structure of each individual. The law of recapitulation claimed that the individual organism, during its development passes through states that correspond to those that occurred during the history of mankind. To sum up, the individual relives the development of the human race from early animal like primitivism, through a period of savagery, to the more recent civilized ways of life that characterize maturity (Muuss, 1975, p. 33). Therefore, Hall described adolescence as a new birth, "for the higher and more completely human traits are now born" (Hall, 1916, xiii). Hall describes this particular aspect of adolescent development (storm and stress) in detail in a chapter of his book on adolescence "Feelings and Psychic Evolution." He saw the emotional life of the adolescent.

Sigmund Freud and the Psychoanalytic Theory of Adolescent Development

Freud paid relatively little attention to adolescent development only to discuss it in terms of psychosexual development. He shared a common idea with that of Hall's evolutionary theory: that the period of adolescence could be seen as phylogenetic. Freud did maintain that the individual goes through the earlier experiences of mankind in his psychosexual development. According to Freud and psychoanalytic theory, the stages of psychosexual development are genetically determined and are relatively independent of environmental factors (Muuss, 1975, p.38). Freud believed that adolescence was a universal phenomenon and included behavioral, social and emotional changes; not to mention the relationships between the physiological and psychological changes, and the influences on the self-image. He also stated that the physiological changes are related to emotional changes, especially an increase in negative emotions, such as moodiness, anxiety, loathing, tension and other forms of adolescent behavior.

Anna Freud's Theory of Adolescent Defense Mechanism

Anna Freud assigns greater importance to puberty as a critical factor in character formation. She also places much emphasis on the relationship between the id, the ego and the superego. She believes that the physiological process of sexual maturation, beginning with the functioning of the sexual glands, plays a critical role in influencing the psychological realm. This interaction results in the instinctual reawakening of the libidinal forces, which, in turn, can bring about psychological disequilibrium. The painfully established balance between ego and id during the latency period is disturbed by puberty, and internal conflict results. Thus, one aspect of puberty, the puberty conflict, is the endeavor to regain equilibrium (Muuss, 1975, p.43).

Anna Freud dealt mainly with deviant or pathological development and paid very little attention to normal sexual adjustment. She described obstacles to normal development:

1) the id overriding the ego - in which she says no trace will be left of the previous character of the individual and entrance into adult life will be marked by a riot of uninhibited gratification of instincts (Freud, 1948, p. 163); and, 2) the ego may be victorious over the id and confine it to a limited area, constantly checked by numerous defense mechanisms.

Among the many defense mechanisms the ego can use, Freud considered two as typical of pubescence: asceticism and intellectualization. Asceticism is due to a generalized mistrust of all instinctual wishes. This mistrust goes far beyond sexuality and includes eating, sleeping, and dressing habits. The increase in intellectual interests and the change from concrete to abstract interests are accounted for in terms of a defense mechanism against the libido. This naturally brings about a crippling of the instinctual tendencies in adult life, and again the situation is "permanently injurious to the individual" (Freud, 1948, p.164).

Anna Freud believes that the factors involved in adolescent conflict are:

- The strength of the id impulse, which is determined by physiological and endocrinological processes during pubescence.

- The ego's ability to cope with or to yield to the instinctual forces. This in turn depends on the character training and superego development of the child during the latency period.
- The effectiveness and nature of the defense mechanism at the disposal of the ego.

Otto Rank's Emphasis on the Adolescent Need for Independence

Otto Rank (1884-1939), a follower of the psychoanalytic school had been completely under the influence of Freudian realism (Rank, 1945, p.209). He then later developed his own theory and began to challenge Freud's notions. Rank saw human nature not as repressed and neurotic, but as creative and productive. He criticized Freud's emphasis on the unconscious as a storehouse for past experiences and impulses. Rank pointed out that the past is of importance only to the degree that it acts in the present to influence behavior. He also places less emphasis on instinctual forces and instinctual behavior. He believed that Freud actually neglected the role of the ego and gave value to it only as a repressive force. Rank wanted to restore the balance of power in the psychic realm (Muuss, 1975, p.47). Rank stated that there must be an examination of the place that adolescent development has in this psychoanalytic theory based on consciousness and 'will'. Sexuality is no longer the strongest determining factor in the developmental process. It has found its counterpart in 'will', which can to some degree, control sexuality. It is during the shift from childhood to adolescence that a crucial aspect of personality development occurs - the change from dependence to independence (Muuss, 1975, p.47). During the latency period, the 'will' grows stronger, more independent, and expands to the point where it turns against any authority not of its own choosing. The actual origin of the 'will' goes further back into the oedipal situation. It is here that the individual will encounter a social will, represented by parents and expressed in a moral code centuries old (Muuss, 1975, p .47).

Erik Erikson's Theory of Identity Development

The core concept of Erikson's theory is the acquisition of an ego-identity, and the identity crisis is the most essential characteristic of adolescence. Although a person's identity is established in ways that differ from culture to culture, the accomplishment of this developmental task has a common element in all cultures. In order to acquire a strong and healthy ego-identity the child must receive consistent and meaningful recognition of his achievements and accomplishments (Muuss, 1975, p.55).

Adolescence is described by Erikson as the period during which the individual must establish a sense of personal identity and avoid the dangers of role diffusion and identity confusion (Erikson, 1950). The implication is that the individual has to make an assessment of his or her assets and liabilities and how they want to use them. Adolescents must answer questions for themselves about where they came from, who they are, and what they will become. Identity, or a sense of sameness and continuity, must be searched for. Identity is not given to the individual by society, nor does it appear as a maturational phenomenon; it must be acquired through sustained individual efforts. Unwillingness to work on one's own identity formation carries with it the danger of role diffusion, which may result in alienation and a lasting sense of isolation and confusion. The virtue to be developed is fidelity. Adhering to one's values contributes to a stable identity.

Kurt Lewin's Field Theory and Adolescence

Kurt Lewin (1890-1947) was a pupil of the early Gestalt school of psychologists at the University of Berlin. He was influenced by Freud's psychoanalytic theory, specifically as it relates to motivation. But Lewin's theory on adolescence is conceptually different from other theories. His theory on adolescent development is explicitly stated in "Field Theory and Experiment in Social Psychology" (1939). His field theory explains and describes the dynamics of behavior of the individual adolescent without generalizing about adolescents as a group. His constructs help to describe and explain, and predict the behavior of a given individual in a specific situation. In a sense, the field theory of adolescence is expressed explicitly and stated more formally than other theories of adolescent development. Field theory has successfully integrated the biological and sociological factors, which are frequently considered contradictory (for example, the nature vs. nurture issue). Lewin makes explicit his position: "the psychological influence of environment on the behavior and development of the child is extremely important" (Lewin, 1935)"psychology in general [is regarded] as a field of biology" (Lewin, 1935).

Lewin's theory of development is of the view that adolescence is a period of transition in which the adolescent must change his group membership. While both the child and the adult have a fairly clear concept of how they fit into the group, the adolescent belongs partly to the child group, partly to the adult group, without belonging completely to either group. Parents, teachers, and society reflect this lack of clearly defined group status; and their ambiguous feelings toward the adolescent become obvious when they treat him at one time like a child and at another time like an adult. Difficulties arise because certain childish forms of behavior are no longer acceptable. At the same time some of the adult forms of behavior are not yet permitted either, or if they are permitted, they are new and strange to the adolescent.

The adolescent is in a state of "social locomotion," since he is moving into an unstructured social and psychological field. Goals are no longer clear, and the paths to them are ambiguous and full of uncertainties--the adolescent may no longer be certain that they even lead to his goals. Such ambiguities and uncertainties are illustrated will by the boy asking or hesitating to ask for his first date. Since the adolescent does not yet have a clear understanding of his social status, expectations, and obligations, his behavior reflects this uncertainty. For example, the adolescent is confronted with several attractive choices that at the same time have relatively impervious boundaries. Driving a car, smoking pot, dropping acid, having sexual relations are all possible goals with positive valence, and thus they become a part of the adolescent's life space. However, they are also inaccessible because of parental restrictions, legal limitations, or the individual's own internalized moral code. Since the adolescent is moving through a rapidly changing field, he does not know the directions to specific goals and is open to constructive guidance, but he is also vulnerable to persuasion and pressure

The self-image of an individual depends upon his body. During the normal developmental process, body changes are so slow that the self-image remains relatively stable. The body image has time to adjust to these developmental changes so that the individual knows his own body. During adolescence changes in body structure, body experience, and new body sensations and urges are more drastic so that even the well-known life space of the body image becomes less familiar, unreliable, and unpredictable. The adolescent is preoccupied with the normality of his body and how his body is perceived by others; he is concerned about and may actually be disturbed by his body image. He spends considerable time studying his own image in the mirror and is concerned about the development of primary and secondary sex characteristics in relationship to age-mates. This is understandable; obviously, the body is especially close to and vital to one's feelings of attractiveness, stability, security, and one's sex role. Negative feelings about one's own body are related to a negative self-concept and may lead to emotional instability that can change one's orientation toward life. Because of these various uncertainties adolescent behavior is characterized by an increased plasticity of personality that can lead to personality changes and even religious conversions (Muuss, 1975, p. 125).

Field theory defines adolescence as a period of transition from childhood to adulthood. This transition is characterized by deeper and far-reaching changes, a faster rate of growth, and differentiation of the life space as compared with the preceding stage of late childhood. The transition is also characterized by the fact that the individual enters a cognitively unstructured region that results in uncertainty of behavior. Transition from childhood to adulthood is obviously a universal phenomenon, since children become mature adults in all societies. However, the shift from childhood to adulthood can occur in different patterns. It can take the form of a sudden shift, such as has been observed in primitive societies in which the puberty rites end childhood and signify the beginning of adulthood

According to Lewin, there are also cultural differences in adolescent behavior. He attributes these differences to several factors: the ideologies, attitudes, and values that are recognized and emphasized; the way in which different activities are seen as related or unrelated (for example, religion and work are more closely related in Mennonite society than in American society as a whole); and, the varying length of the adolescent period from culture to culture and from social class to social class within a culture. Moreover, the degree to which the child group and the adult group are differentiated in a given culture has far-reaching consequences for adolescent behavior. The more clearly they are separated, the more difficult the transition (Lewin, 1942, as cited in Muuss, 1975, p.130).

Roger Barker's Somatopsychological Theory of Adolescence

Roger Barker and others expanded and elaborated Lewin's theory of adolescent development in "Somato Psychological Significance of Physical Growth in Adolescence" (1953, as cited in Muuss, 1975, p.130). He uses the field theory to illustrate the effects of physiological changes on behavior during adolescence. According to Barker body dimensions, physique, and endocrinological changes occur at an accelerated speed during adolescence as compared to the preadolescent years. As a result, some corresponding psychological situations occur.

First, "new psychological situations" arise during adolescence; and second, experiential psychological situations will take place in which "overlapping of the psychological field" occurs. According to Barker, in the US, the child group is clearly separated from the adult group, for whom different forms of behavior are accepted. Children have a social position equivalent to that of a minority group; this increases the difficulty of moving from one group to the other. The possibility of moving from one social group to the other is determined informally by one's physique: looking like an adult makes it easier to get adult privileges (Muuss, 1975, p.132).

Allison Davis: Adolescence and Socialized Anxiety

Allison Davis defines "socialization" as the process by which an individual learns and adapts the ways, ideas, beliefs, values, and norms of his culture and makes them part of his personality. He sees development as a continuous process of learning socially acceptable behavior by means of reinforcement and punishment. Acceptable and unacceptable behavior are defined by each society, or its socializing agents, the subgroups, social classes, or castes. Cultural behavior is acquired through social learning. Understanding the effects of social learning on adolescents is the crucial issue in Davis' theory (Muuss, 1975, p. 139). Socialized anxiety serves as a motivating and reinforcing agent in the socialization process: it brings about "anticipation of discomfort" and becomes a behavior-controlling mechanism. It is Davis' hypothesis that the effective socialization of adolescent behavior is dependent upon the amount of adaptive or socialized anxiety that has been implanted in an individual. If an individual's socialized anxiety becomes strong enough, it will serve as an impetus toward mature, responsible, normal behavior. It is implied that if socialized anxiety is too weak or too strong, the attainment of mature behavior is less likely (Muuss, 1975, p. 140).

The goals of socialization differ from culture to culture and from social class to social class within a culture. Social anxiety becomes attached to various forms of behavior depending upon the expectations, values, and definition of what is normal in a given social class. As an example, the case is given that the middle class child acquires moral values, needs, and social goals different from those of the lower or upper class child. Furthermore, since the middle class is more concerned with normality, success, morality, and status, the amount of socially instilled anxiety is greater than in the other classes.

It is the characteristic of middle-class youth that his social anxiety increases with the onset of adolescence, since he faces new developmental and behavioral tasks, such as preparation for work and heterosexual adjustment. Furthermore, since the middle class is more concerned with normality, success, morality, and status, the amount of socially instilled anxiety is greater than in the other classes. It is characteristic of middle-class youth that his social anxiety increases with the onset of adolescence, since he faces new developmental and behavioral tasks, such as preparation for work and heterosexual adjustment. Furthermore, as he becomes increasingly aware of his own social needs - having prestige, friends, being accepted by the peer group, relating to the opposite sex - he becomes more sensitive to social cues and social pressures. Since he depends greatly upon social acceptance, prestige, and status, his social anxiety increases. This produces an increased striving for socially desirable goals. "Adolescents with a strongly developed social anxiety, therefore, usually strive for the approved social goals most eagerly and learn most successfully" (Davis, 1944, p. 208, as cited in Muuss, 1975, p. 140).

Robert Havighurst's Developmental Tasks of Adolescence

According to Robert Havighurst, developmental tasks are defined as skills, knowledge, functions, and attitudes an individual has to acquire at a certain point in his or her life; they are acquired through physical maturation, social expectations, and personal efforts. Successful mastery of these tasks will result in adjustment and will prepare the individual for the harder tasks ahead. Failure in a given developmental task will result in a lack of adjustment, increased anxiety, social disapproval, and the inability to handle the more difficulty tasks to come (Muuss, 1975, p. 141).

Each task is the prerequisite for the next one. For some of these tasks, there is a biological basis and consequently, there is a definite time limit within which a specific task must be accomplished. The inability to master a task within its time limit may make later learning of that task more difficult, if not impossible. Therefore, Havighurst believes there is a "teachable moment" for many developmental tasks. Through its socializing agents and method of reinforcement and punishment, society attempts to help the individual learn those developmental tasks at their proper age levels (Muuss, 1975, p.142).

The developmental tasks for adolescence (from about 12 to 18 years) are:

- Accepting one's physique and accepting a masculine or feminine role.
- New relations with age-mates of both sexes.
- Emotional independence of parents and other adults.
- Achieving assurance of economic independence.
- Selecting and preparing for an occupation.
- Developing intellectual skills and concepts necessary for civic competence.
- Desiring and achieving socially responsible behavior.
- Preparing for marriage and family life.
- Building conscious values in harmony with an adequate scientific world-picture.

(Havighurst, 1951, pp.30-55, as cited in Muuss, 1975, p.142)

There seems to be little disagreement on the fact that adolescence is a transition period between childhood and adulthood. Two theorists, however, Bandura (1964) and Hollingsworth (1928) believed that human development is a continuous process not divided into stages. They believed that if adolescence has become a transition period for some individuals in our society, social conditions are responsible, not some intrinsic aspect of human development. Lewin describes the adolescent as the marginal man and some other theorists seems to support his view. Coleman (1961), in his book, "The Adolescent Society", speaks of a teen-ager subculture, the adolescent society, which includes a large segment of the population for a fairly long period of time. The transitional period is more noticeable if the child and adult groups are well defined, as they are in America today. This transition requires a re-evaluation of one's relationship to the external world, to the social world, and to one's own internal, psychic world. (Muuss, 1975). It is observed that theorists such as Sherif (1947), Erikson (1959), and Friedenberg (1959), consider adolescence as the crucial period for the formation of the mature ego. Mead's research seems to support this idea as she states: "In most societies adolescence is a period of reexamination, and possible reorientation" (Mead, 1949, p.361, as cited in Muuss, 1975, p.267).

Piaget (1947) sees adolescence as a "decisive turning point...at which the individual rejects, or at least revises his estimate of everything that has been inculcated in him, and acquires a personal point of view and a personal place in life." There also is agreement by theorists that, during adolescence, the time perspective expands, and past and future assume greater importance and become clearly differentiated. Piaget says that the adolescent can build theories and reflect beyond the present and, according to Muuss (1975, p.267), this corresponds to a more definite planning of vocational activities, preparation for marriage, and the establishment of more specific and lasting life goals, including the need for achieving emotional and economic independence. During adolescence, the unreality or fantasy level decreases in importance and is more clearly distinguished from reality. Childlike play also decreases as obligations, responsibility, and social expectations increase (Muuss, 1975, p.267).

According to Muuss (1975), most theories postulate an important transitional phase of early adolescence between ten and fourteen years for girls and eleven and fifteen or sixteen for boys. What theorists no longer agree on is that there is a universal period of storm and stress. There is new evidence that adolescence is not typically a time of storm and stress but that experience a relatively stress-free period (Bandura, 1964; Offer, 1969).

Cultural Anthropology and Adolescence: Margaret Mead

There are several studies by cultural anthropologists that shed light on adolescent development. The contributions of one great anthropologist, Margaret Mead, gave us much insight into perspectives on adolescent development in a cultural context. Mead wrote 2 books that relevant to a discussion of adolescence: Coming of Age in Samoa (1950) and Growing Up in New Guinea (1953). The first book is devoted entirely to the adolescent period.

Coming of Age in Samoa is an empirical field study; it uses anthropological methodology, but does not contain an explicitly stated theory of adolescent development. But, Ruth Benedict in "Continuities and Discontinuities in Cultural Conditioning" (1954), provides an explicit theory of development from a cultural anthropological point of view which she relates directly to Mead's study of adolescence in Samoa. It is from these theoretical writings that a systematic statement about the importance of cultural factors in the developmental process was summated. "Cultural relativism" - a term more appropriate to the earlier than later writings of Mead - contributes new and important ideas to the understanding of the phenomenon of adolescence. It emphasizes the importance of social institutions and cultural factors in human development and describes the rituals of pubescence as well as adolescent experiences in primitive societies.

In the past, there was a period which both Erikson and Mead called a "psychological moratorium," an "as if" period during which youth could tentatively experiment without being asked to show “success" and without final emotional, economic, or social consequences. The loss of such a period of uncommitted experimentation, during which youth can find itself makes it difficult to establish ego-identity. As a substitute, for psychological identity, youth utilizes peer group symbols to establish a semi-identity of deprived and/or semi criminal groups. According to Mead, even education has become functional and "success" oriented. Consequently, the goals and values of adolescents are directed toward success, security, immediate gratification of desires, conformity, and social acceptance with little room for experimentation, idealism, utopianism, and personal martyrdom. Mead states that "failure to adopt our educational and social system...may be held responsible for some of the sense of self-alienation, search for negative identities, and so forth, characteristic of this present group of young people" (Mead, 1961, p.49, as cited in Muuss,1975, p.111).

Mead does advocate greater freedom for the adolescent and less conformity to family, peer and community expectations to allow the adolescent to realize his creative potential. She states, "We can attempt to alter out whole culture, and especially our child-rearing patterns, so as to incorporate within them a greater freedom for and expectation of variations" (Mead, 1951, p.185 as cited in Muuss, 1975, p.112). Mead also criticizes the American family for its too intimate organization and its crippling effect on the emotional life of the growing youth. She believes that too strong family ties handicap the individual in his ability to live his own life and make his own choices. She suggests that "it would be desirable to mitigate, at least in some slight measure, the strong role which parents play in children's lives, and so eliminate one of the most powerful accidental factors in the choices of any individual life" (Mead, 1950, p.141 as cited in Muuss, 1975, p.112) and, Muuss (1975) points out that even though Mead objects to the pattern of the American family that produces conformity and dependency in its children, she considers the family a tough institution and demonstrates that it is nearly universal. Mead knows of no better way to produce wholesome individuals than through a tolerant family system in which "father says 'yes' and mother says 'no' about the same thing" (Mead, 1947, p.330 as cited in Muuss, 1975, p.112), and in which the adolescent can disagree with his parents without a resulting loss of love, self-respect, or increase of emotional tensions.

Ruth Benedict's theory of continuities and discontinuities in cultural conditioning has important educational implications according to Muuss (1975). Our educational practices at home as well as in school should emphasize continuity in the learning process so that the child becomes conditioned to the same set of values and behavior in childhood that will be expected from him in adulthood. The child should be taught nothing that he will have to unlearn in order to become a mature adult. Changes in behavior, often constituting a discontinuity, are expected as the individual moves from elementary to high school, from college into the labor market, and from denial of sexuality before to sexual responsiveness following the wedding.

Adolescence and Mental Health

Being a teenager is hard. Teenager would be under stress to be liked, do well in school, get along with family, and make big decisions. Most of these pressures, and worrying about them is normal. But feeling very sad, hopeless or worthless could be warning signs of a mental health problem. Mental health problems are real, painful, and sometimes severe.

- Often feel very angry or very worried
- Feel grief for a long time after a loss or death
- Think your mind is controlled or out of control
- Use alcohol or drugs
- Exercise, diet and/or binge-eat obsessively
- Hurt other people or destroy property
- Do reckless things that could harm you or others

Mental health problems can be treated. Help can be done by parents, school counselors, or health care providers.

Adolescent Mental Health Issues

Many mental health problems emerge in late childhood and early adolescence. Recent studies have identified mental health problems - in particular depression, as the largest cause of the burden of disease among young people.

Poor mental health can have import effect on the wider health and development of adolescents and is association with several health and social outcomes such as higher alcohol, tobacco and illicit substances use, adolescent pregnancy, school dropout and delinquent behaviours. There is growing consensus that healthy development during childhood and adolescence contributes to good mental health and can prevent mental health problems.

Teenage is an important period which is inevitable in the life of every individual. If Mental Health Issues exist among Adolescents and they are not given much attention and hence untreated they become worse in future, some problems can be turned into to life long risks as well as other issues could get converted to age specific risks.

Over the course of life, if a person experience mental health problems, then his thinking, mood, and behavior could be affected. Many factors contribute to mental health problems, including:

- Biological factors, such as genes or brain chemistry
- Life experiences, such as trauma or abuse
- Family history of mental health problems

Mental health problems are common but help is available. People with mental health problems can get better and many recover completely.

Doctors have pondered the connection between our mental and physical health for centuries. Until the 1800s, most believed that emotions were linked to disease and advised patients to visit spas or seaside resorts when they were ill. Gradually emotions lost favor as other causes of illness, such as bacteria or toxins, emerged, and new treatments such as antibiotics cured illness after illness.

More recently, scientists have speculated that even behavioral disorders, such as autism, have a biological basis. At the same time, they have been rediscovering the links between stress and health. Today, we accept that there is a powerful mind-body connection through which emotional, mental, social, spiritual, and behavioral factors can directly affect our health.

Mind-body medicine focuses on treatments that may promote health, including relaxation, hypnosis, visual imagery, meditation, yoga, and bio-feedback.

Over the past 20 years, as per WHO 2014 reports mind-body medicine has provided evidence that psychological factors can play a major role in such illnesses as heart disease, and that mind-body techniques can aid in their treatment. Clinical trials have indicated mind-body therapies to be helpful in managing arthritis and other chronic pain conditions. There is also evidence that one can help to improve psychological functioning and quality of life, and may help to ease symptoms of disease.

Good mental health is a sense of wellbeing, confidence and self-esteem. It enables us to fully enjoy and appreciate other people, day-to-day life and our environment. When we are mentally healthy we can:

- form positive relationships
- use our abilities to reach our potential
- deal with life's challenges

A few tips for positive mental health are:

- talk about or express your feelings
- exercise regularly
- eat healthy meals
- get enough sleep
- spend time with friends and loved ones
- develop new skills
- relax and enjoy your hobbies
- set realistic goals
- talk to your health professional

Figure 1

Figure on Aspects Affecting the Mental Health of Children and Adolescents

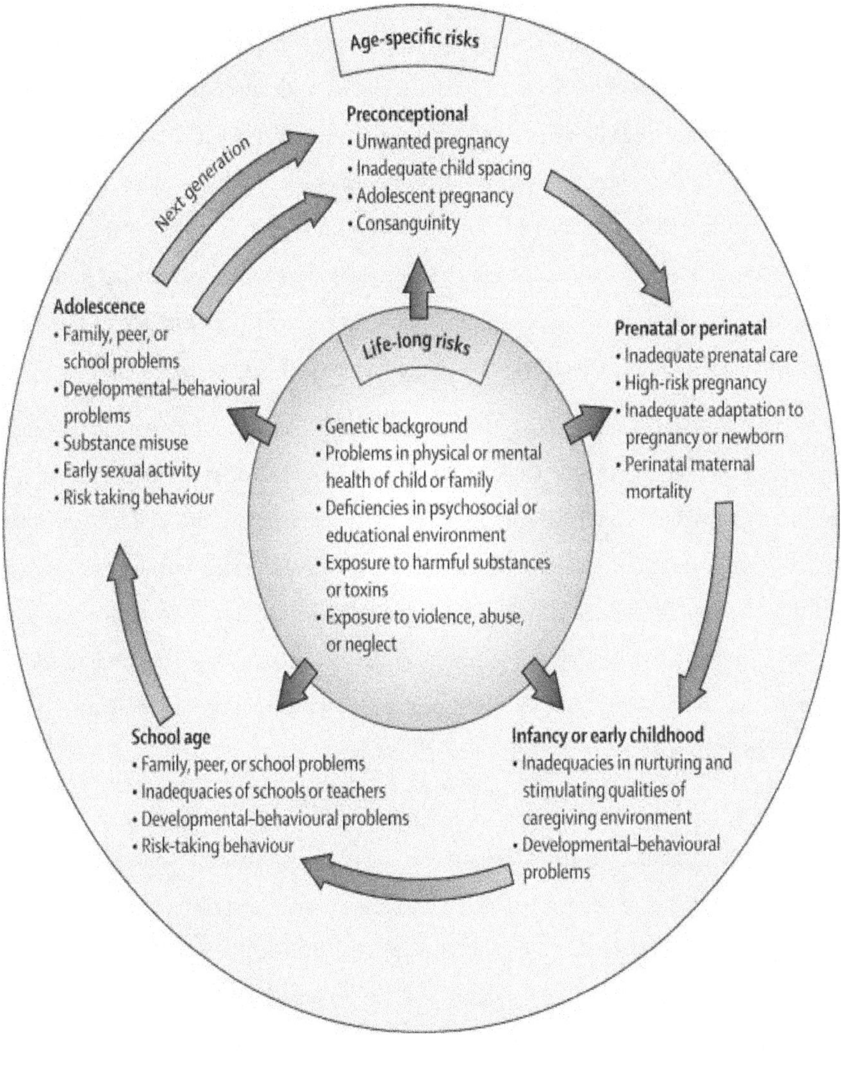

Need of the Study

. Mental health problems in young people can lead to tragic consequences, including suicide, substance abuse, inability to live independently, involvement with the correctional system, failure to complete high school, lack of vocational success, and health problems.

There is a lack of mental health services for children and adolescents. Families that are poor, are people of color, or have children with other disabilities or health concerns have an especially difficult time getting services that would identify, prevent or treat mental health problems. Children and adolescents with mental health problems are usually involved with more than one agency or service system, including mental health, special education, child welfare, juvenile justice, substance abuse, and health. However, no agency or system usually takes responsibility for coordinating their care or prevents them from falling through the cracks and not getting needed services.

As adolescents are assets of every country, mental health problems of adolescents can make adverse and drastic damage for the development of every country. Mental health issues affect children, adolescents, and their families as well as schools, communities, employers, and the nation as a whole. The present study is meant to analyse the different aspects and the relation of personality traits and home environment in the mental health of adolescent girls. The results of the present study could be used to adopt ways to increase mental health of adolescent girls and to find out the problems from family and other home environment which affects the mental of girls

Conclusion

Peace of mind is a natural condition, and is available to everyone, when one's mindset become free of depression, anxiety, excessive stress and worry, addictions, and other psychological problems and will be more able to live life to the fullest. Mental health strengthens and supports individual's ability to have healthy relationships and to make good life choices, to maintain physical health and well-being and also to handle the natural ups and downs of life.

CHAPTER II

REVIEW OF LITERATURE

Introduction

A literature review is a text of a scholarly paper, which includes the current knowledge including substantive findings, as well as theoretical and methodological contributions to a particular topic. Review of related literature is a crucial aspect in the planning of a new study. The related studies on the chosen topic carried by research workers at various levels are called review of literature. It is a key step in research process and works as a guide which enables one to perceive the lacuna in the concerned field of research. A literature review is an evaluative report of information found in the literature related to the selected area of study. The review should describe, summarise, evaluate and clarify this literature. It should give a theoretical base for the research and help the author to determine the nature of your research.

Reviews on Mental Health of Adolescents

Lisa and Alan (2009) made an attempt to study on the leisure, boredom and adolescent risk behavior and it was published in the journal of child and adolescent mental health. A systematic review of literature was conducted and it was evident that the experience of leisure, boredom is influenced by a variety of different factors, not least of which is the environment or context within which adolescents are situated. The review focuses attention leisure, boredom as a factor contributing to risk behavior in adolescents.

Geetha and Vijayalakshmi (2006) made an attempt in their study to find out the impact of emotional maturity of adolescent in their stress and self confidence. Sample of the study consisted of 105 adolescents studying in XI and XII standards at Dharwad city, Karnataka state, India. The findings revealed that adolescent with high emotional maturity had significantly high stress and self confidence, when compared to those with low emotional maturity.

Keyes and Corey (2006) conducted a study on mental health in adolescents. The second wave of child development supplement of the panel study of income dynamics, in which a comprehensive set of subjective well being items were administrated to a sample of 1,2,3,4 youth ages 12-18. Moderate health was the most prevalent diagnosis among youth ages 15-18. Findings suggested the importance of positive health in future research on adolescent development.

In 2005 researchers investigated the psycho social correlates of identity formation in adolescent boys and girls. For this purpose, a sample of 200 adolescents aged 18-20 years was selected from the various school of Amritsar. The samples were administered with various tools to measure identity status, emotional autonomy, family environment, well-being, intellectual capacity and personality. Result suggested identity formation was positively linked with health and congenial home environment, emotional autonomy well-being and personality (**Damanjit and Suninder, 2005**).

Young (2004) in his study has pointed out that mental health issues interfere with student success more than ever before. Young brought to light how mental health issues could affect the success of students in the present scenario more than ever before. He also indicates that the rate of depression among college students rose almost five percent in just the years with 38% of these student are antidepressant medication and over are undergoing through therapy. In the study "College of the Overwhelmed" the researchers wrote on the campus mental crisis and what to do about it. The paper confirms that a rising number of students are coping with depression anxiety and other major mental health challenges. They suggested that in addition to the normal developmental concerns of traditional aged college student today students are pressured to get good grades, hold down jobs and become involved in college life, coping with the financial realities a college education is also extremely stressful for many. For some minority, international first generation or immigrant Students College may mean dealing with new forms of discrimination, a lack of role models family expectations and challenges in daily living activities. (**Kadison and Digeronimo, 2004**)

Gallaher et al. (2000) had remarked in their study that almost all directors counselling centres surveyed and noted the increase in the number of students entering into college campuses who are already taking psychotropic medications. In a portrait of today's college student, **Levine and Cureton (1998)** opines that generally students are coming to educational institutions more damaged and overwhelmed with anxiety than those of previous years.

Walker et al. (1998) conducted a study promoting adolescent mental health in primary care: the study states that mental health problems in adolescent can be prevented by early detection and treatment.

Discussion on Stated Reviews

The above mentioned studies on Mental Health of Adolescent points out that among those influencing factors, environment plays vital role or situation where individuals are located. Certain studies states that adolescent with high emotional maturity had significantly high stress and self-confidence, when compared to those with low emotional maturity. Research reviews confirms that a rising number of students are coping with depression anxiety and other major mental health challenges. Findings suggested the importance of positive health in future research, on adolescent development. Research review suggested that the identity formation was positively linked with health and congenial home environment, emotional autonomy, wellbeing and personality. Researchers opine that generally students are coming to educational institutions more damaged and overwhelmed with anxiety than those of previous years. Some studies states that mental health problems in adolescent can be prevented by early detection and treatment.

Reviews on Mental Health of Adolescent Girls

A crucial element of all research degrees is the review of relevant literature. So important is this chapter that its omission represents a void or absence of a major element in research. **Coverdale and Long (2015)** have conducted a study on Emotional wellbeing and mental health: an exploration into health promotion in young people and families. Promoting mental health and emotional wellbeing (EWB) in children and young people (YP) is vitally important for their psycho-social development. Critical review of the literature reveals a dearth of research that has explored the perspective of the child, adolescent or adult in this concept, with much research being intervention focused and promoted at crisis level. The current study aims to address this gap in understanding of young persons' and parents' perspectives.

Nagaraja et al. (2015) have conducted a study on the Prevalence of Depression among College Students of Kolar District, Karnataka State. Nursing College is recognized as a stressful environment that often exerts a negative effect on the academic performance, physical health and psychological wellbeing of the student. This study aimed to assess the prevalence of depression and its associated factors among nursing students of Kolar district. Materials and methods: A Stratified random sample of 430 students was assessed using separate questionnaire by investigators. Association between depression and class of studying, age group, social factors like family problems, family history of depression and staying away from home were analyzed. The prevalence of depression was significantly more among those with family problems and family history of depression. Prevalence of depression is highly prevalent among nursing students in this area. Our findings point to the importance of broad screening and psychiatric counseling of this vulnerable population.

Researchers have conducted a study on the Barriers to Mental Health Treatment for Children and Adolescent: A Systematic Review. Despite the higher prevalence of mental health problem among children and adolescent, the rate of mental health services utilization among this group is still low. Among small number of children and adolescents attended mental health treatment, many of them tend to prematurely terminate the treatment offered. This systematic review aims to provide an overview reported barriers to mental health treatment for children and adolescents from the perspectives of parents or caregivers. Attitudinal barrier especially believed that nothing could help is one of the main barriers to mental health treatment for children and adolescent. School-based program could improve children's and adolescent's mental health status by reducing the barriers **(Siti et al., 2015).**

Cetin et al. (2014) have conducted another study on Evaluation and Follow-Up of Gender Identity and Sexual Orientation Problems in Adolescents: Four Female Cases. Gender Identity Disorder (GID) is defined as a continuous and severe discomfort of an individual's biological sex and gender identity role, a strong desire to be a member of the other gender and the presence of a strong identification with the opposite gender. A mutual interaction between biological factors, cultural characteristics and values occur during the construction of the sense of gender identity. The treatment of psychological problems comorbid with gender identity disorders, maintaining school attendance in formal education system, the integrity of family and their supportive attitudes towards their children are significant for the follow up process and preventive psychological health.

A study on systematic review of online youth mental health promotion and prevention interventions was conducted by **Clarke (2014).** The rapid growth in the use of online technologies among youth provides an opportunity to increase access to evidence-based mental health resources. The aim of this systematic review is to provide a narrative synthesis of the evidence on the effectiveness of online mental health promotion and prevention interventions for youth aged 12-15 years. Searching a range of electronic databases, 28 studies conducted since 2000 were identified. Eight studies evaluating six mental health promotion interventions and 20 studies evaluating 15 prevention interventions were reviewed. The results from the mental health promotion interventions indicate that there is some evidence that skills-based interventions presented in a module-based format can have a significant impact on adolescent mental health, however, an insufficient number of studies limits this finding.

Dusunen (2014) have conducted a study on The present study examined the direct and indirect relationships between parent-adolescent conflict, self-esteem, and depression symptoms. Participants were 338 (150 male, 188 female) adolescents aged between 14–18 attending public high schools. Participants completed a questionnaire that included measures of parent-adolescent conflict, self-esteem, and depression symptoms. Findings provided evidence of direct effects of parent-adolescent conflict on depression symptoms and indirect effects of mother adolescent conflict on depression symptoms through self-esteem. Specifically, results indicated that mother adolescent conflict were positively and directly related to self-esteem, and indirectly related to depression through self-esteem.

A study was conducted on Promoting mental health and wellbeing for a young person with a mental illness: parent occupations. Parenting is a critical and complex occupational role, requiring different occupations and abilities depending on the developmental stage and specific characteristics of each child. The way parents respond to mental illness can have an important impact on young people. This research demonstrates the breadth of the mental illness related occupations parents employ and provides a framework for understanding their complexities. It highlights the need to establish an evidence base for various mental illness related occupations so that parents can have more knowledge and thus confidence in these critical occupations **(Honey et al., 2014)**.

A research study was conducted on the evaluation of quality of life, self-esteem, peer relationship and anger levels in adolescents with acne at an university hospital: a case control study done by **Ozden et al. (2014).** Acne vulgaris occurs mostly during adolescence, a time when social and physical changes occur at the maximum level, and identity formation is a matter. In adolescence, when the perfect look is idealized, and in societies where physical attractiveness is important, acne can be a devastating disease. This study aims to evaluate the peer relationship, self-respect and anger level of 81 adolescents who presented to a dermatology outpatient clinic with acne in comparison with age- and sex-matched, healthy adolescents without any skin diseases. There was no significant relationship between quality of life and gender and severity of acne. Significant correlations were detected between quality of life and trait anger and anger-in (respectively; $r=0.397$, $r=0.346$). There were no significant differences in terms of peer relationship, anger levels, anger style, Piers Harris total score and its subscale scores as intellectual and school status, behavior, conformity, popularity and social appreciation, anxiety, happiness and satisfaction between the acne and the control groups. However, the self-esteem on physical appearance was significantly lower in acne group than in the control group.

Dhanalakshmi (2013) assessed self concept, anxiety and mental health among adolescent boys and girls. The results indicated that gender differences exist on all three variables. Adolescent girls indicated better self concept and mental health compared to boys. Self concept was positively correlated to anxiety while mental health was negatively correlated to anxiety.

Dubey and Srivastava (2013) studied parental factors, achievement motivation and performance of adolescents. High performing adolescents reflected higher achievement motivation in comparison to low performance group of students. Parental approval emerged as the most significant predictor of achievement motivation and performance followed by resources made available by parents, parental encouragement and parental pressure. The high performance group girls were more future oriented with high level of aspiration as their expected and achieved scores are less discrepant. They expected more and achieved less than their expectations. These findings imply that in order to improve children's education, parental approval warrants the future orientation. Adolescents in modern society spend a remarkable amount of their time with their peers. They spend most of each weekday with their peers while at school, and a vast majority also see or talk to their friends in the afternoon, evening and over the weekend. Experience in the peer group is also vital for the development and expression of autonomy. The process of developing more mature and more independent relationships with parents is accompanied by the establishment of more mature.

Kaur and Singh (2013) assessed emotional intelligence of adolescent children in relation to their locus of control. Results indicated that on emotional intelligence, male and female students differ significantly with male students being more emotionally intelligent. The males were more internally oriented than the females. No significant differences were found between the internally and externally oriented students on all components of emotional intelligence whether males or females. Despite popular stereotypes of storm and stress in the adolescent's family, scientific studies indicate that there is very little emotional distance between young people and their parents. Although some adolescents and their parents have serious interpersonal problems, majority of adolescents feel close to their parents, respect their parent' judgement, feel that their parents love and care about them and have a lot of respect for their parents as individuals. Parents are likely to see these as issues of right and wrong – not in moral sense, but as a matter of custom and convention. Adolescents, in contrast, are likely to define the issues as matters of personal choice. Studies of family interaction suggest that early adolescence is a time during which young people begin to try to play a more forceful role in the family but parents may not yet acknowledge the adolescents' input. As a result, young adolescents may interrupt their parents more often but have little impact. By middle adolescence, however, teenagers act and are treated more like adults. They have more influence over family decisions, but they do not need to assert their opinions through interruptions and similarly immature behavior.

Jane et al. (2012) conducted study on Adolescent Mental Health, Behavior Problems, and Academic Achievement. Prior research on the association of mental health and behavior problems with academic achievement is limited because it does not consider multiple problems simultaneously. Combinations of problems involving substance use were especially consequential. Our results demonstrate that the social consequences of mental health problems are not the inevitable result of diminished functional ability but, rather, reflect negative social responses. These results also encourage a broader perspective on mental health by demonstrating that behavior problems heighten the negative consequences of more traditional forms of distress.

Mason et al. (2012) have conducted a research on A systematic review of the role of school-based healthcare in adolescent sexual, reproductive, and mental health. To evaluate the effects of school-based healthcare services on the sexual, reproductive and mental health of adolescents. The Services had to target adolescents and focus on sexual, reproductive and mental health outcomes. Outcomes included knowledge and use of hormonal contraception, condom use, emergency contraception, receipt of testing for sexual transmitted disease/infection, care related to pregnancy and HIV prevention, pregnancy rate, age at first sexual experience, suicide attempt and ideation, substance use and educational outcomes. The evidence was severely limited and equivocal on the effectiveness of school-based healthcare for sexual, reproductive and mental health outcomes in adolescents.

Kwako et al. (2011) determined emotional intelligence (EI) and social support differ in traumatized depressed patients when compared with controls. The result indicates that traumatized depressed participants exhibited lower total emotional intelligence, because of reduction in strategic EI ability, as well as lower levels of social support compared with the control group.

Stuart and Mavis (2011) have conducted a study on Physical activity and mental health in children and adolescents. To synthesize reviews investigating physical activity and depression, anxiety, self-esteem and cognitive functioning in children and adolescents and to assess the association between sedentary behavior and mental health by performing a brief review. Reviews on physical activity and cognitive functioning have provided evidence that routine physical activity can be associated with improved cognitive performance and academic achievement, but these associations are usually small and inconsistent. Primary studies showed consistent negative associations between mental health and sedentary behaviour. Association between physical activity and mental health in young people is evident, but research designs are often weak and effects are small to moderate. Evidence shows small but consistent associations between sedentary screen time and poorer mental health.

Ay dim and Kamilebehar (2010) examined whether strategies theory predict adolescents mental health to a significant level. The study was conducted on a sample of 119 students (61 females and 58 males) age range from 14 to 17 years. Results explained that the most powerful predictor of the mental health is the ACE (Active/effective Contact with the Environment) strategy of coping with stress. The results also illustrate that as the adolescent's level of stress coping strategies decrease, their level of psychological symptoms increases.

Leicester (2010) have conducted a study on Antisocial Personality Disorder Treatment, Management and Prevention (2010) The guideline on Antisocial Personality Disorder, commissioned by NICE and developed by the National Collaborating Centre for Mental Health, sets out clear, evidence- and consensus-based recommendations for staff working in health and social care and the criminal justice system on how to treat, manage and prevent antisocial personality disorder. It includes a review of interventions in children and young people with conduct disorder, risk assessment and management; organisation and experience of care; and a range of interventions for adults with antisocial personality disorder, including psychological interventions, treatment for comorbid disorders, therapeutic communities and pharmacological interventions. The book also contains a useful overview of antisocial personality disorder, including ethical considerations.

Morsunbul (2010) have conducted a study on Approaches/Models Which Explain Development during Adolescence: Results of Approaches/Models In Terms of Adolescent Mental Health. Youths show great effort to construct their identity during adolescence. A lot of models/approaches have been proposed by taking Erikson's psychosocial developmental theory as the basis. The aim of this review was to investigate approaches / models which were developed in light of Erikson's theory. According to the results of the review, some models/approaches were proposed which deal with propositions of Erikson's identity development theory. Discussion: It can be said that adolescents who experience actively exploration process are healthier in terms of mental health.

Nada and Tatjana (2010) have conducted a study on Age, Gender and Disorder Related Personality Characteristics of Pediatric Patients Measured by Eysenck Personality Questionnaire. The study of personality is important not only for psychology and related disciplines, but also in clinical practice. The starting point in this article is Eysenck theory of personality, based primarily on genetics and physiology which corresponds to the temperament. Main categories of temperament for Eysenck are extroversion vs. introversion, neuroticism vs. stability and psychoticism vs. socialisation. Total number of examinees was N = 216 (90 girls, 126 boys). It was shown that EPQ is good choice for differentiation of the main personality traits in children which help in the assessment procedure measuring extroversion, neurotic and psychopathologic traits which is useful for planning treatment options.

Catharine et al. (2010) studied intelligence in early adulthood and subsequent hospitalization for mental disorders. The results indicate that lower intelligence is a risk factor for the whole range of mental disorders and for illness severity.

Gupta and Kumar (2010) studied the relationship of mental health with emotional and self-efficacy among 200 (100 male and 100 female) college students from Kurukshetra University. The result indicates that emotional intelligence and self-efficacy are positively related with mental health. It also revealed that male students were better than female students in term of mental health, emotional intelligence and self -efficacy.

Jafar and Siti (2010) study examined whether, spiritual intelligence (SI) and emotional intelligence (EI) can be considered as predictor for mental health. The participants in the study were 247 High school students (124 male and 123 female) in the age range of 14-17 years old, at the Gorgan City, north of Iran. The result indicates that mental health can be influenced by spiritual intelligence and emotional intelligence. In addition, the moderated effect of age on the relationship of spiritual intelligence and emotional intelligence with mental health was not found.

Junger and Kampes (2010) studied the cognitive ability and self- control in relation to dietary habits, physical activity and body weight in adolescents. The result indicates that adolescents scoring high on the cognitive ability test have healthier dietary habits and engage more often in physical activity.

Martins et al. (2010) studied a comprehensive meta-analysis of the relation between emotional intelligence and health and showed that emotional intelligence is associated with better health. The weighted average association with mental (r 0.36) and psychosomatic health (r 0.33) was higher, than the association with physical health (r 0.27).

Noradilah et al. (2010) determines the association between several selected demographic characteristics and the mental health status of 1467 youngsters studying in Malaysian Public Universities. The findings of the study indicate that a majority of undergraduate students exhibits a healthy mental state while a majority has shown some mental health concerns. Further in the present study results of the analysis of variance also showed that the student's mental health condition differed in terms of ethnicity, academic field and year of the study.

Shabani and Hassan (2010) investigated the link of intelligence with mental health in 247 Iranian of high school students of 8 schools (124 Boy and 123 Girl). The results indicate that there is significant relationship of intelligence with mental health.

Gladys and Frank (2009) examined the 599 Taiwan college students to study the relationships of physical activity, emotional intelligence and health. The results indicate that the physical activity is an effective way to improve the physical, psychological as well as emotional health of college students.

Glaser et al. (2009) examined the relationship between total intelligence quotient (IQ) score at age 8 years, and depressive symptoms at 11, 13, 14 and 17 years. The result showed that IQ at age 8 years was inversely associated with depressive symptoms at age 11 years, but the association changed direction by age 13 and 14 years when a higher IQ score was associated with a higher risk of depressive symptoms. This change in IQ effect was also found in relation to pubertal stage. At age 17 years, however, sex-specific differences emerged. Whilst the risk effect of higher childhood IQ scores for depressive symptoms declined in females, and some analyses even supported an inverse association by age 17 years, it persisted in males.

Karestan and Terrie (2009) studied the association between childhood IQ and adult mental disorders .The result indicates that lower childhood IQ was associated with increased risk of developing schizophrenia spectrum disorder, adult depression, and adult anxiety. Thus, many patients who seek mental health treatment may have lower cognitive ability.

Knutson et al. (2009) studied the association between childhood IQ and adult mental disorders. The result indicates that lower childhood IQ was associated with increased risk of schizophrenia, adult depression and anxiety.

Simonton and Song (2009) studied the relationships among achieved eminence, IQ, early physical and mental health, and achievement domain. The correlation and regression analyses showed, for these 282 individuals, that eminence is a positive function of IQ and that IQ is a positive function of mental health and a negative function of physical health, implying an indirect effect of physical and mental health on eminence.

Siti et al. (2009) examined the degree of relationship between self-esteem, stress and loneliness with depression among 1,407 secondary school students (age range 13 to 17 years). The findings of the study showed that self-esteem, loneliness and stress have a moderating significant relationship with depression, further results show that stress emerged as the strongest predictor of adolescent's depression.

Suldo and Elizabeth (2008) in a study investigated the relationship among coping, stress and mental health in 139 students participated in an International Baccalaureate (IB) high school Diploma program. The results of the study indicated that students in an IB program perceive significantly general education peers and learn those specific coping styles that are differently associated to student's mental health outcomes. Furthermore, findings also shown that coping styles (specially, positive appraisal and anger) moderate the influence of internalizing symptoms of psychopathology and stress on global life satisfaction of students.

Meral (2008) have conducted a study on TAF Preventive Medicine Bulletin. The use of digital technology, including computers, cell phones, computer games, and so on, most recently, on-the-go for recreational purposes, has increased among our youth over the past 15 years. Children and adolescent between the ages of 8 to 18 years spend an average of 5-6 hours per day using information and communication technologies. It is a useful progress because of the increase of internet usage which is unlimited, uncontrolled and uninhibited and easiness which arrival all sorts of to information's or persons but this state can cause to some important negative results too. The computer games, the internet explores is gradually estrange from social life the children and adolescent. In this paper, has been mentioned to negative effect of internet usage, computer games on mental health of children and adolescents.

Wessel et al. (2008) studied the relationship between emotional- social intelligence (ESI) and each of leadership, caring and moral judgment. The result indicates that positive relationship between ESI and leadership and ESI may be an important construct in caring but ESI was not related to moral judgment.

Kumar et al. (2007) studied that high intelligence is associated with better mental health and less fatigue.

Montes and Augusto (2007) studies conducted with nurses or nursing students has shown that emotional intelligence is a skill that minimizes the negative stress consequences. Hierarchy regression analysis pointed out that clarity and emotional repair are predictors of social support, and emotional repair is the main predictor of mental health.

Schembri et al. (2006) results revealed that high intelligence to be associated with positive well-being; and deficits in intelligence with poor mental health.

Schutte et al. (2006) investigated the relationship between emotional intelligence and health. The result of meta-analysis on the responses of 7898 participants found that higher emotional intelligence was associated with better health.

De Moor et al. (2006) examine whether regular exercise is associated with anxiety, depression and personality in a large population - based sample as a function of gender and age. The findings suggest that regular exercise is cross-sectionally associated with lower neuroticism, anxiety and depression and higher extroversion and sensation seeking in the population than non- exercises. These differences were modest in size, but very consistent across gender and age.

Liu et al. (2005) studied the mental health condition of the only child: A study of urban and rural high school students in China. The sample of the study consisted of 632 students (mean age=17.2 years). The results of the study showed that urban only child experienced significantly higher social depression and neurotic, trait anxiety, interpersonal dependency and perceived stressors as well as lower love awareness of family than did urban non-only children. Low love awareness also predicted perceived stressors which resulted in negative mental health.

The relationship between parent adolescent communication including adolescent's depression, self-esteem and shyness was explored. The results of the study showed that, the quality of four family patterns differed significantly with each other. Amongst all four patterns of families the best one was pluralistic family, the second best was laissez faire families, third best was consensual families and fourth best was protective families. Moreover results also revealed that parent adolescent communication quality and communication pattern have different predictive effects on depression, self-esteem and shyness of adolescents. (**Sun et al., 2004**)

Jung (2003) studied "Adolescent self-concept and heath into adult hood". He found that self-concept tends to be low among girls compared with boys. A strong self-concept had a positive long-term effect on girl's self-perceived health.

Diener et al. (2002) have conducted a study on the Personality, Culture, and Subjective Well-Being: Emotional and Cognitive Evaluations of Life. Subjective Well-Being (SWB), people's emotional and cognitive evaluations of their lives, includes what lay people call happiness, peace, fulfillment, and life satisfaction. Personality dispositions such as extraversion, neuroticism, and self-esteem can markedly influence levels of SWB. Although personality can explain a significant amount of the variability in SWB, life circumstances also influence long-term levels. Cultural variables explain differences in mean levels of SWB and appear to be due to objective factors such as wealth, to norms dictating appropriate feelings and how important SWB is considered to be, and to the relative approach versus avoidance tendencies of societies. Culture can also moderate which variables most influence SWB. Although it is challenging to assess SWB across societies, the measures have some degree of cross-cultural validity. Although nations can be evaluated by their levels of SWB, there are still many open questions in this area.

Leventhal et al. (2000) has conducted a study on the effects of neighborhood residence on child and adolescent outcomes. Provides a comprehensive review of research on the effects of neighborhood residence on child and adolescent well-being. The 1st section reviews key methodological issues. The third section identifies 3 pathways (institutional resources, relationships, and norms/collective efficacy) through which neighborhoods might influence development, and which represent an extension of models identified by C. Jencks and S. Mayer (1990) and R. J. Sampson (1992). The models provide a theoretical base for studying neighborhood mechanisms and specify different levels (individual, family, school, peer, community) at which processes may operate. Implications for an emerging developmental framework for research on neighborhoods are discussed.

Discussion on Stated Reviews

The above discussed reviews on Mental Health of Adolescent Girls suggested that the social consequences of mental health problems are not the inevitable result of diminished functional ability but, rather, reflect negative social responses. Some studies demonstrate that behavior problems heighten the negative consequences of more traditional forms of distress. Reviews on physical activity and cognitive functioning have provided evidence that routine physical activity can be associated with improved cognitive performance and academic achievement. Some studies states that there is association between physical activity and mental health in young people is evident. Results explained that the most powerful predictor of the mental health is the ACE (Active/effective Contact with the Environment) strategy of coping with stress. Emotional repair is the main predictor of mental health. Certain studies suggested that regular exercise is cross-sectionally associated with lower neuroticism, anxiety and depression and higher extroversion and sensation seeking in the population than non- exercises.

Reviews on Mental Health and Personality of Adolescent Girls

The word 'personality' refers to the pattern of thoughts, feelings and behaviour that makes each of us the individuals that we are. These affect the way we think, feel and behave towards ourselves and others. We don't always think, feel and behave in exactly the same way – it depends on the situation we are in, the people with us and many other things. But we mostly tend to behave in fairly predictable ways. Personality may influence the mental health of adolescent girls.

The mentioned reviews suggests that **Davila et al. (2016)** studied on Navigating romantic relationships in adolescence/young adulthood and finds that it is a normative developmental task that can be both pleasurable and challenging for youth.. This chapter reviews the literature on the associations between psychopathology and youth romantic relationships and experiences. We focus particularly on internalizing and externalizing disorders, for which the bulk of the literature exists. We also cover eating disorders and attention-deficit/hyperactivity disorder (ADHD) as well as other disorders and issues of comorbidity. Following the reviews of specific disorders and symptoms, we review the emerging literature on psychopathology and same-sex relationships among youth. We then address key peer and family contexts in which psychopathology and skills for romantic relationships are developing, and we discuss the intergenerational transmission of psychopathology and romantic dysfunction.

Sally et al. (2012) states that depression is common in young people, has a marked negative impact and is associated with self-harm and suicide. Preventing its onset would be an important advance in public health. To determine whether psychological or educational interventions, or both, are effective in preventing the onset of depressive disorder in children and adolescents. Standardized, validated, and reliable rating scales of depression, or both, were included. Two authors independently assessed studies for inclusion and rated their quality. Sample sizes were adjusted to take account of cluster designs and multiple comparisons. Fifty-three studies including 14,406 participants were included in the analysis. Sixteen studies including 3240 participants reported outcomes on depressive diagnosis. The persistence of findings suggests that this is real and not a placebo effect. Psychological and educational interventions can help in preventing depression in children and adolescents. Depressive disorder is common and has a major impact on the functioning of young people. The aim of this review was to assess the effectiveness of programmes designed to prevent its onset.

Pérez and Cumsille (2011) analyzed the way in which adolescents' temperamental characteristics interact with parental control to shape adolescent decision making development. A sample of high-school Chilean adolescents (N = 391) answered a self-report questionnaire that included measures of behavioral autonomy (the extent to which adolescents make decisions in personal and prudential domains), parental behavioral and psychological control, and temperamental characteristics. A path analysis model indicated that adolescents' anger-frustration had a direct association with decision-making in the personal and prudential domains; fearfulness had an inverse association with adolescent decision-making, but only in the prudential domain. Perceived psychological control was associated with adolescents' reduced decision-making autonomy in the personal domain, while perceived behavioral control was associated with less adolescent autonomy in both personal and prudential domains. Additionally, a moderation effect was found such that the association of parental behavioral control on decision-making in the prudential domain was dependent on the adolescent fearfulness level.

Dhanya and Rekha (2011) attempted to compare the Self –concept, Educational and occupational aspirations, general expectation and general performance of adolescents from the community living with their families and those in the orphanages. They found that adolescent girls living with family had a secure, warm, supportive environment where they had more care, advice and encouragement from their parents. On the other hand adolescent girls living in orphanage were not blessed with a good living environment, which in turn affected their self-concept, aspirations, general expectation and performance aspects.

Ruth and Ulrich (2011) examined the development of self-esteem in adolescence and young adulthood. For this purpose a sample was taken from the young aduh section of the National Longitudinal Survey of Youth, which includes eight assessments across a 14 year period of a national probability sample of 7,100 individual's age range 14 to 30 years. The results of the study indicated that level of self-esteem increases during adolescence and continue to increase more slowly in young adulthood, where males and females did not differ in their self-esteem trajectories. The findings also revealed that during adolescence Hispanics had lower levels of self-esteem than Blacks and Whites, but the self-esteem of Hispanics subsequently increases more strongly, so that at age 30 Blacks and Hispanics had higher level of self-esteem than Whites. However, at each age emotionally stable, conscientious and extroverted individuals experienced a higher level of self-esteem than less conscientious individuals, emotionally unstable and introverted. Moreover, at each age level low risk taking behaviour, high sense of mastery and better health predicted higher self-esteem.

Ahadi and Basharpoor (2010) studied the relationship between sensory processing sensitivity, personality dimensions and mental health in a sample of University of Mohaghegh Ardabili students. The results revealed that ease of excitation was positively correlated to neuroticism and mental health (physical problems, anxiety, disorder in social functioning and depression) and negatively related to extraversion. Aesthetic sensitivity was positively related to neuroticism, openness to experience, conscientiousness and anxiety. Low sensory threshold was also positively related to neuroticism, physical problems, anxiety and mental health. The results also revealed that sensory processing sensitivity can explain considerable variances of personality traits and mental health.

Bimal and Ashok (2010) studied "Sociometric status in relation to personality characteristic and Intelligence of High school students". The sample of 124 male students divided into three groups of 45, 42 and 37 was selected by using purposive sampling technique from one district of Orissa. The findings were (1) there exists significant positive relationship between sociometric status derived from the sociometric criterion and personality factors A, E, F and Q (2) In case of 14 personality factors measured by High-School Personality Questionnaire, factors B, D, E, G, H, O and Q2 are simple measures. The remaining personality factors have emerged to be complex measures. (3) Positive personality traits have been found to be more important than negative ones in making a person popular.

Cloninger and Zohar (2010) studied the personality and the perception of health and happiness on the sample of 1102 volunteer representatives of the Sharon area of Israel. The finding suggests that self-directedness was strongly associated with all aspects of well-being regardless of interactions with other dimensions. Cooperativeness was strongly associated with perceived social support, and weakly with other aspects of well-being, particularly when Self-directedness was low. Self-transcendence was strongly associated with positive emotions when the influence of the other character dimensions was taken into account. Personality explained nearly half the variance in happiness and more than one-third of the variance in wellness.

Grace (2010) investigated the relationships between big five personality traits (i.e. neuroticism, extraversion, agreeableness, openness to experience and conscientiousness) and psychological resilience among n397 Caribbean adolescents. The results of the study revealed a significant positive relationship between the personality traits (i.e. conscientiousness, agreeableness, openness to experience, and extraversion) and psychological resilience, while neuroticism was negatively correlated with psychological resilience. Furthermore, personality traits jointly contributed 32% variance in psychological resilience and this was found to be statistically significant with conscientiousness being the most excellent predictor while agreeableness, neuroticism and openness to experience were other significant predictors, however adolescents psychological resilience was not predicted by extraversion one of the personality trait.

Meenakshi (2010), studied "Personality needs and Academic Achievement of Sr. Secondary students". A sample of 120 students of X class was selected from 5 schools in Ghaziabad city. She used Meenakshi Personality Inventory. She found that need-achievement, need dominance, need-nurturance and need-endurance are positively and significantly related to students' academic achievement. It is found that some students have low achievement and the cause is the low level of related need.

Namita and Lipsamayee (2010) studied "Self-concept, Personality type and Ethical values among Adolescents". Data were collected from 60 adolescents (30 boys and 30 girls). They found that adolescent girls were found to be more ethical than the boys of their age. There was no gender difference with regard to self-concept and Personality type.

Lockenhoff et al. (2009) examined the association between five- factor personality domains and facets and spirituality/religiousness as well as their joint association with mental health in a diverse sample of 112 people living with HIV. Spirituality/ religiousness showed stronger associations with conscientiousness, openness, and agreeableness than with neuroticism and extraversion and both personality traits and spirituality/religiousness were significantly linked to mental health, even after controlling for individual differences in demographic measures and disease status. Personality traits explained unique variance in mental health above spirituality and religiousness.

Joshanloo and Nosratabadi (2009) investigated the discriminatory power of personality traits (i.e. neuroticism, extraversion, openness, agreeableness and conscientiousness) in discriminating among the levels of mental health continuum using a sample of Iranian university student. The findings of the study revealed that students with different levels of mental health condition differ significantly on four of the five traits of personality that is extraversion, neuroticism, conscientiousness and agreeableness.

Abbott et al. (2008) studied individual differences in personality influence the occurrence, reporting and outcome of mental health problems across the life course. Women who were more socially outgoing (extrovert) reported higher well-being on all dimensions. Neuroticism was associated with lower well-being on all dimensions. The effect of early neuroticism on midlife well-being was almost entirely mediated through emotional adjustment defined in terms of continuities in psychological/psychiatric distress. The effect of extraversion was not mediated by emotional adjustment, nor attenuated after adjustment for neuroticism.

Lincoln (2008) studied that an individual's personality traits may mediate the relationship between social support and mental health. The findings of the study revealed that students with different levels of mental health condition differ significantly on four of the five traits of personality that is extraversion, neuroticism, conscientiousness and agreeableness.

Korotkov (2008) studied a sample of 706 adults to measure if personality moderates the relationship between stress and health behaviour. The findings of the study revealed that students with different levels of mental health condition differ significantly on four of the five traits of personality that is extraversion, neuroticism, conscientiousness and agreeableness.

Ram (2008), did "A Study of Extra vertive and Neuroticism Tendencies of popular, Neglected and Rejected Adolescents Belonging to Different Localities". The present study was conducted on the X class students studying in various government and private co-education institutions located in urban and rural areas. Sample consisted of 1691 students. Hindi version of H.J Eysenck's Personality Inventory prepared by S.S Jalota and S. D. Kapoor was used as a tool. The researcher found that the popular students in boys as well as girls groups and in urban as well as rural groups were found more extroversive in their behavior than the neglected and rejected students.

Osterberg et al. (2007) studied to assess early determinants of idiopathic environmental intolerance (IEI), contributing to an integrated model for the development of idiopathic environmental intolerance (IEI). The findings of the study revealed that students with different levels of mental health condition differ significantly on four of the five traits of personality that is extraversion, neuroticism, conscientiousness and agreeableness.

Shipley et al. (2007) examined the influence of neuroticism and extraversion on all-cause and cause-specific mortality over 21 years after controlling for risk factors. The result showed that after controlling for several risk factors, high neuroticism was significantly related to risk of death from cardiovascular disease. The effect of neuroticism on death from cardiovascular disease may be mediated by socio demographic, health behaviour, and physiological factors. Extraversion was protective of death from respiratory disease.

Benjamin (2006) examined the associations between five factor model of personality traits and mental health and analyses that higher neuroticism score was associated with worse perceived health and a lower extraversion score was associated with worse perceived health.

Lung (2006) conducted a study to examine the personality traits and mental health among Taiwanese military students with adjustment disorder. Among 641 students from two military high schools, 43 had a diagnosis of adjustment disorder. Differences between students with adjustment disorder and those without adjustment disorder were statistically significant in terms of their premorbid personality and mental health. Different kinds of school discipline appear to be a precipitating factor for adjustment disorder; however, neurotic, introvert, and psychotic traits appear to be predisposing factors for adjustment disorder.

Goodwin et al. (2006) studied the association between major depression, neuroticism, and self-reported allergy among adults in the community. The result indicates that among adults in the community, major depression was associated with a significantly increased likelihood of allergy. Higher level of neuroticism was also significantly associated with increased likelihood of allergy.

Hooker (2006) examined the influence of personality on mental and physical health of spouse caregivers and to determine whether there were differences in such influences depending on disease context. The disease contexts compared were Alzheimer's disease (AD) and Parkinson's disease (PD; with no coexisting dementia)- both chronic, degenerative diseases of later life. The result indicates that personality had significant direct and indirect effects on mental health and significant indirect effects on physical health. As predicted, Alzheimer's disease (AD) caregivers had significantly worse mental health than PD caregivers; however, AD caregivers had better physical health than PD caregivers.

Jylha and Isometsa (2006) investigated the relationship of the personality dimensions of neuroticism and extraversion to the symptoms of depression and anxiety in the general population. The result indicates that neuroticism correlated strongly with symptoms of depression and anxiety and somewhat with self-reported lifetime mental disorder. Extroversion correlated negatively with symptoms of depression, anxiety, and self -reported lifetime mental disorder.

Kendler (2006) examined the nature of association between neuroticism and extroversion and the risk for major depression .The result indicates that neuroticism strongly associated with major depression and extroversion were weakly and inversely related to major depression.

McWilliams et al. (2006) investigated the relationship between several personality constructs and the use of outpatient mental health services. The results revealed that personality traits play a role in treatment seeking behaviors for mental health problems over and above the presence of psychiatric disorders alone.

Sanz et al. (2006), studied "Goals and personality of Adolescents". A sample of 1179 adolescents (565 girls and 614 boys) age between 15 and 19 years was studied. Researcher used situational personality Questionnaire and Goals for adolescents Questionnaire. Researcher found that to a great extent, Personality factors – Adjustment, Emotively, Superiority, Independence and sociability- Predict goals pursued. And also he investigated the influence of personality factors in the value allotted by adolescents to various groups of goals.

Sangeeta (2006) studied the relationship between introversion - extroversion and mental health on 600 boys studying in tenth standard in high and higher secondary school of Jammu city. The results indicate that extroversion tendencies enhance the mental health where as introversion tendencies deteriorate mental health.

Tyrer and Mulder (2006) studied the management of severe and complex personality disorders in community mental health services. The result indicates that severe personality disorders have a negative impact on the outcome of most psychiatric disorders.

Scholte et al. (2005), studied "Adolescent personality types and subtypes and their psychosocial Adjustment". A sample of 3,284 Dutch adolescent boys and girls was studied. They found that the personality subtypes were associated with very distinctive adjustment patterns.

Srivastava (2004) studied mental health and personality adjustment among optimistic and pessimistic students. Results indicated a significant difference between optimistic and pessimistic students with respect to mental health and personality adjustment. In addition, a significant relationship was found between mental health and personality of pessimistic students but no such relationship was found for optimistic students. Besides the family environment, many socio-cultural factors in a child's physical environment affect his emotional, social, cognitive and personality development.

The main objective of the study was to analysze the affect of socio-culturally depriving factors on the mental health status of Indian adolescents. Results revealed that adolescents of both groups differed significantly on four out of five scales of mental health status inventory except on the scale of expression. Results confirmed the hypothesis that socio-cultural deprivation has an adverse effect on the mental health of the adolescent. The mental health status of young females is worth exploring. Girls, during their schooling years, have many conflicts and anxieties due to their physical and emotional growth. Studies have revealed that there is a reversal of sex ratio of stress manifestation between boys and girls due to conforming to traditional roles. Hence the girls manifest neurotic anxiety over the state of ambivalence and confusion during their adolescence phase. They manifest more personality problems such as shyness, jealousy, sensitivity and physical complaints.

Sharma (2003) conducted a study with the objective to develop a scale to measure life skills and to assess the levels of life skills in adolescents of a secondary school at Kathmandu. A descriptive, cross sectional survey of adolescents from class VIII, IX, and X of a public co-educational econdary school of Kathmandu was done with the help of self-administered questionnaires prepared in English and translated into Nepali. Focus Group Discussions consisting of boys only, girls only and a mixed group comprising of one student from each section of each class were conducted to confirm the results of the study. All the data obtained from the questionnaire survey were edited, coded and entered into EPI info Version 6. Mother's education was significantly associated with Increased level of life skills in adolescents (P=.001). It was concluded that most of the teachers were not aware of the concept of life skills. Maternal education was significantly associated with higher life skill levels in adolescents. Connectedness and family support were other important factors influencing the level of life skills in the adolescents.

Weiqun (1999) studied stress and mental health condition of secondary school students in Shanghais the effects of collectivism and Guanxi. The sample of the study consists of 2,986 respondents aged 15 to 19 years. Findings showed that stress and mental health problems experienced by adolescents in urban China were mainly socially oriented. Further perceived stress found to be negatively related to positive well-being also positively related to psychological distress. However, the collective behavioural tendency was found to be inversely related to positive well-being but negatively related to psychological distress. In some social context was found to play a significant role in shaping adolescents development in urban China. Final results show that the resources identified such as collectivism and guanxi have a significant influence on mental health outcome of adolescents.

Discussion on Stated Reviews

The above discussed reviews on mental health and personality of adolescent girls states that a moderation effect was found such that the association of parental behavioral control on decision-making in the prudential domain was dependent on the adolescent fearfulness level. Studies shows that ease of excitation was positively correlated to neuroticism and mental health and negatively related to extraversion. Some reviews revealed a significant positive relationship between the personality traits (i.e. conscientiousness, agreeableness, openness to experience, and extraversion) and psychological resilience, while neuroticism was negatively correlated with psychological resilience. Studies also suggested that extroversion tendencies enhance the mental health where as introversion tendencies deteriorate mental health.

Reviews on Mental Health and Home Environment of Adolescent Girls

Bandy and Ottoni (2012) investigated whether family structure transition and low income are risk factors in the development of pro-social behavior. Models of young adults' prosocial behavior charitable giving and volunteering were estimated as functions of their family structure and income during the stages of childhood. Participants were a representative sample of 1011 American young adults. In the full sample, family structure transition during adolescence was negatively associated with subsequent charitable giving in young adulthood. Low income during adolescence was negatively associated with both giving and volunteering in young adulthood. European-American young men also exhibited a negative association between family structure transition during adolescence and subsequent volunteering. The results did not seem to describe African-American young adults. Keeping this qualification in mind, the results suggested that adolescence is a sensitive stage in the development of charitable giving and volunteering.

emotionally expressive; democratic with regard to discipline, input, and decision making; close but not enmeshed; higher in their level of parent-adolescent communication and family ideals; and lower in external locus of control.

Chawla Anita (2012) aimed to test the relationship between family environment and academic achievements. The participants included in the study were two hundred students i.e. 100 boys and 100 girls, randomly selected from the 9th standard of Marathi medium schools of Nasik City. Family Environment Scale by Dr. Harpreet Bhatia and Dr. N.K. Chadha (1993) was used for the purpose of data collection. Second semester (yearly) marks of 9th standard were taken. Data analysis was done by using Pearson correlation coefficient. Findings of the study revealed that family environment score was positively correlated with the academic achievement of the students.

Leung and Shek (2012) based on the responses of 275 Chinese adolescents experiencing economic disadvantage in Hong Kong, the relationships between family processes (including perceived parenting style, parental control, family functioning, and parental sacrifice for children's education) and psychosocial competence were examined in the study. Results showed that parenting style, parental control, family functioning, and parental sacrifice for children's education were positively related to adolescent psychosocial competence. Regression analyses indicated that family functioning, maternal control, and paternal sacrifice for children's education were significant predictors of psychosocial competence of adolescents experiencing economic disadvantage. The theoretical and practical implications of the findings were discussed.

Shuster et al. (2012) examined interrelations among cultural values, parenting practices, and adolescent aggression using longitudinal data collected from Chinese adolescents and their mothers. Adolescents' overt and relational aggression were assessed using peer nominations at Time 1 (7th grade) and Time 2 (9th grade). Mothers reported endorsement of cultural values (collectivism and social harmony) and parenting practices (psychological control and inductive reasoning) at Time 1. While controlling for Time 1 adolescent aggression, maternal collectivism and social harmony indirectly and longitudinally linked to adolescent aggression through maternal parenting practices.

Deepshikha and Bhanot (2011) conducted a study at Kumarganj, Faizabad District of Eastern Uttar Pradesh. The purpose of the study was to assess family environment of adolescent girls and its impact on their socio-emotional adjustment. One hundred adolescent girls of age group between 17-18 years comprised the sample of the study. Family Environment Scale (FES) and Adjustment Inventory for School Students (AISS) were administered. Data was analyzed in terms of percentage and multiple regression analysis. The statistical analysis revealed that all the eight family environment factors, viz. cohesion, expressiveness conflict, acceptance and caring, independence, active-recreational orientation, organization and control together showed significant role in socio-emotional and educational adjustment of adolescent girls.

Oliver et al. (2011) examined in a long-term longitudinal study, the relation between aspects of adolescents' family context representing a supportive and intellectually stimulating environment and subsequent qualities of transformational leadership in every day leaders in early adulthood. In addition, they examined one pathway through which this link occurs. Specifically, they sought to determine whether the relation between positive family functioning and transformational leadership was mediated through functioning and transformational leadership mediated by self-concept, controlling for socioeconomic status. When parents provided a stimulating and supportive environment, adolescents reported a more positive general self-concept, which subsequently related to transformational leadership qualities in adulthood. These findings represented the first prospective data that support the relation of family environment in childhood to transformational leadership in adulthood.

Enrique et al. (2010) analysed the relationship between psychosocial quality of family context and the cognitive development of a sample of 551 children of school age. The data were gathered at school and at home in two waves, when the children were 5 (T1) and 8 (T2) years old, respectively. In T1, three factors related to quality of family context were obtained: absence of conflict, child -family adjustment, and sociability. Two factors of cognitive development were obtained in T1 and T2. In T1, associations were found between all three factors and cognitive development. In T2, associations were found between the quality of family context and cognitive development. Cognitive development in T2 was predicted by the absence of conflict T1 factor, with a negative association. Children who were exposed to more conflicts in T1, and who scored higher on the HOME scale in T2, were found to have improved their cognitive development scores over time in comparison with their group.

Acharya and Joshi (2009) intended to study the influence of parental education level on achievement motivation of adolescents. A total of 200 intermediate students belonging to parents having four levels of education (high school, intermediate, graduation and post graduation) were administered Deo-Mohan achievement motivation scale. The result indicated that parental education level influences the achievement motivation in academic area. Higher the level of parental education, better the achievement motivation in academic area. Other areas were not found to be significantly influenced by the level of fathers' and mothers' education.

Delva et al. (2009) in a cross sectional survey assessed the psychological well-being and socio-economic hardship of orphan and non- orphan children in Conakry, Guinea. The study included 133 orphan and 140 non-orphan children. Multiway analysis of variance and multiplelogistic regression models were used to measure the association. The result showed that the psychological well-being score was significantly lower among orphan children than non- orphan children. The study recommended for sustainable and holistic approaches to ensure the psychological and socio- economic stability of orphans and other vulnerable children.

Kaur et al. (2009) attempted to explore academic achievement and home environment as correlates of self-concept in a sample of 300 adolescents. The results of the study revealed self-concept to be positively correlated with academic achievement, though not significantly so. A significantly positive relationship of home environment components of protectiveness, conformity, reward, and nurturance with self-concept was revealed, thereby meaning that use of rewards and nurturance from parents should be done for positive self-concept development among adolescents. However, the correlation of social isolation, deprivation of privileges and rejection components of home environment was significantly negative with self-concept among adolescents indicating that for positive self-concept development among adolescents, there should be less or no use of social isolation, deprivation of privileges and rejection. The study had implications for educationists and parents as well.

Kaur and Singh (2009) investigated the relation between home environment, self-concept, and academic achievement in 2,297 14–15 yr old Koreans. Results showed that over the 4 samples, self-concept was a mediating variable between home environment and academic achievement. Results did not support the commonly held view that home environment exerts direct effects on academic achievement. Social status indicators had indirect effects on self-concept via family psychological characteristics. Academic self-concept affected academic achievement more strongly than did presentation-of-self or social self-concept.

Drozdz and Pokorski (2007) evaluated the relationships among perceived parental attitudes and domains of social competence in late adolescents. Forty boys and 40 girls, all aged 18, representing a population sample of high school second graders were examined. Self-report data were collected using questionnaires of parent-child relations and of social competence. Analyses detected a significant association between the maternal loving or protective attitude and competence in interpersonal relations in the combined sample of adolescents. However, gender was a moderator of this general relationship. Maternal control fostered their sons' interpersonal relations, and no such relationship was observed toward daughters. Adolescents' behavior was somehow less influenced by fatherly control. The findings were in line with the concept of familism as a dominant form of family organization, but implicate constraints in parental sentiments whose overly expression may backfire and do more harm than good in other domains of social competence of adolescents, such as assertiveness and performance during social exposure. The study might contribute to future research on how parenting style shapes adolescent social outcomes.

Ganesh and Magdalin (2007) compared children from disrupted families institutionalized) and children from non-disrupted families in terms of academic stress and perceived problems. A sample of 80 boys, 40 from disrupted families (institutionalized) and 40 from non- were as follows: i) Mooney's Problem Checklist, and ii) Rajendran's Academic Stress Questionnaire. Results indicated that children from non-disrupted families have higher academic stress than children from disrupted families. Similarly, with regard to perceived problems, significant difference was found between the two major groups in the following sub-scales: Health and Physical Development, Finance,

Living Conditions and Employment, Social- Psychological Relations, Personal Psychological Relations, Courtship, Sex and Marriage, Adjustment to School Work, Future: Vocational and Educational.

Martinez and Garcia (2007) studied the relationship of parenting styles with adolescents' outcomes within a sample of Spanish adolescents. The results showed that Spanish adolescents from indulgent households have the same or better outcomes than adolescents from authoritative homes. Parenting was related with two self-esteem dimensions—academic and family—and with all the self-transcendence and conservation values. Adolescents of indulgent parents showed highest scores in self-esteem whereas adolescents from authoritarian parents obtain the worst results. In contrast, there were no differences between the priorities given by adolescents of whereas adolescents of authoritarian and neglectful parents, in general, assigned the lowest priority to all of these values.

Aishwarya and Arora (2006) investigated the perceived parental behaviour and its relationship with academic school success and academic competence. The sample comprised of 500 High School students (250 male and 250 female). The subjects were administered Adolescent's Perception of Parental Behaviour Questionnaire (APPBQ) developed by Arora, Sinha and Lakshmi. A School Success was assessed by marks obtained in High School Board Examination. Academic Competence Scale was also developed by Arora and Lakshmi. Results of the study revealed that parental acceptance and encouragement scores were positively related with academic school success and academic competence scores. However, parental control (psychological and behavioral) showed negative relationship with academic success and competence. Parents who were perceived as being more acceptant and using less restrictive and hostile psychological control tended to have adolescents with higher academic success and competence.

The effect of motivation, family environment, and student characteristics on academic achievement of 388 high school students (193 males and 195 females) from Abu Dhabi District, United Arab Emirates (UAE) was done by **Halawah (2006).** A Likert-type instrument was used that consisted of three parts (scales) to measure students' level of motivation, parental influences, and students' characteristics, while academic achievement was measured using student's GPA. Calculations were also breakdown by gender to assess differences between male and female students. Students' mean level of motivation was less than the means of parental influence and student's characteristics. No gender differences were observed on the variables measured by the instrument. Correlations between each of motivation, family environment, student characteristics and academic achievement were small and practically not significant. Remarkably high correlation value was observed between motivation and students characteristic. The highest correlation value was observed between family environment and students' characteristics.

Slicker et al. (2005) surveyed at a large, mid-south university in the USA, 660 university freshmen (mean age = 17.9 years; 68.2% female; 86.5% non-Hispanic white) regarding their perceptions of their parents 'parenting behaviors and their perceptions of their own life-skills development. Simultaneous regression results indicated that parental responsiveness significantly predicted life-skills development in all four domains even when age, gender, and socioeconomic status were taken into account; whereas, parental demandingness was not a significant predictor in any of the four domains of life-skills development. The results of this study suggested that positive life-skills development in older adolescents is related to having been reared by a parenting style high in responsiveness.

Arali and Rathna (2004) studied "Influence of family environment on emotional competence of adolescents" with a sample of 120 adolescents. Family environment scale of Bhatia and Chadda and Emotional Competency scale by Bhardwaj and Sharma were used as tools. They found that majority of adolescents' perceived average cohesion, expressiveness, conflict, acceptance and caring, active recreational orientation organization and control except independence. Majority of adolescents were average in all competencies and emotional competence in general except encouragement of positive emotional competence.

The importance and role of regard for parents (i.e., how important parents are regarded) for psychosocial competence, as indicated by self-esteem and susceptibility to antisocial peer pressure. Participants were 555 Singapore adolescents in 4 secondary levels (equivalent to Grades 7-10). Results showed that regard for parents was positively related to psychosocial competence, being positively associated with self-esteem and negatively associated with antisocial susceptibility. More interesting, regard for parents was found to have a role in 2 well-established relations between parental practices and psychosocial competence. Regard for parents moderated the relation between parental support and self-esteem (the relation being stronger when regard for parents was high) and mediated the relation between parental monitoring and antisocial susceptibility. These results suggested a need to consider regard for parents for a better understanding of the parent-adolescent dynamics in adolescent psychosocial competence **(Sim, 2000)**.

Mzobanzi and Mboya (1996) investigated the perceived family and social, school environments and their relationships to self-concept of African adolescents. A total of 1,192 secondary school students participated in the study. The findings of the study indicated that perceived parental behaviours were associated with family relation, general school, emotional stability and physical appearance, also relations with peers, global self-concepts and health. Perceived teachers behaviours were associated with family relations, health, general school, global self-concepts and emotional stability.

Abraham (1985) studied the relationship of psycho-social factors with the mental health status of a sample of 880 PUC students. The results of the study revealed that adjustment and other psycho-social factors (need for belongingness, need for acceptance and need for love etc.) were related to the mental health status of the students.

Discussion on Stated Reviews

The review on mental health and home environment of adolescent girls shows that Findings of the study revealed that family environment score was positively correlated with the academic achievement of the students. Results of studies shows that parenting style, parental control, family functioning, and parental sacrifice for children's education were positively related to adolescent psychosocial competence. A significantly positive relationship of home environment components of protectiveness, conformity, reward, and nurturance with self-concept was revealed, thereby meaning that use of rewards and nurturance from parents should be done for positive self-concept development among adolescents. Results of certain study indicated that children from non-disrupted families have higher academic stress than children from disrupted families.

Reviews on Home Environment and Personality Variables Affecting the Mental Health of Adolescent Girls

The literature reviews on the cumulative reviews of the variables like home environment and personality traits affecting the mental health of adolescents states that **Deb et al. (2015)** have studied and examined relationships among home environment, parents' personality and mental health of adolescents with a focus on adjustment, anxiety, self-concept and self-confidence. A group of 370 adolescents were interviewed using a semi-structured questionnaire and three psychological tests; subjects were selected following a two-stage sampling technique. Participation of the adolescent students in the study was voluntary. Results indicate that parental care was associated with high self-confidence while parental pressure associated with high anxiety. Fathers' "friendliness" associated with low emotional adjustment and high self-concept while mothers' short-temper associated with high anxiety. Disturbed families contributed to adolescent anxiety, inability to share personal problems, parental interference in personal affairs and academic pressure. Parental traits were found to negatively influence mental health, e.g., anxiety, adjustment, self-concept and self-confidence. Findings suggest a need for expanding school guidance and counseling capacity to assist parents and adolescents with developmental tasks.

Wray-Lake and Flanagan (2012) assessed factors related to Social Trust (ST) in 11–18 year olds with survey data collected over two years from 1150 U.S. adolescents and their mothers. Adolescents' ST in year 1 and their reports of a positive neighborhood climate predicted ST one year later. Adolescents' reports of family practices were stronger predictors of their ST than were mothers' reports. Regression analyses revealed different factors predicting changes in ST for three adolescent age groups: With ST at T1 and background factors controlled, democratic parenting boosted ST for early- and middle-adolescents. Adolescents' reports that parents encouraged compassion for others boosted ST for middle- and late adolescents, and parental cautions about other people taking advantage diminished ST among middle adolescents. Results suggested that the disposition to trust others is formed, in part, by what adolescents hear from parents about their responsibilities to fellow human beings and by modeling of democratic parenting.

Ashurst et al. (2009) studied the psychosocial experiences of late adolescents coping with parental cancer using a developmental systems framework and grounded theory methods. Results suggested three primary psychosocial developmental influences, including multilevel influences (individual, familial, and extra familial risk and protective factors), coping strategies to maintain control, and responses to uncertainty and anticipatory grief. Identity and intimacy were the two most salient psychosocial tasks. The central unifying concept of resilience was the primary psychosocial developmental outcome that resulted from coping with parental cancer during late adolescence. This finding illuminated the need to expand the focus in youth development research and practice to include positive developmental outcomes that can result from coping with life crises during adolescence.

Estevez et al. (2008) examined the influence of family and classroom environments on the development of particular individual characteristics, including level of empathy, attitude to institutional authority and perceived social reputation, and the role these characteristics may in turn play in school aggression. Participants were 1319 adolescents aged 11–16 (47% male) drawn from state secondary schools in Valencia (Spain). Since previous studies suggest that these variables may contribute differentially to aggressive behaviour depending on adolescent gender, two different mediational structural models were calculated, variables considered in the structural equations tested and pointed out different paths for boys and girls. Overall, the findings suggested that a positive family environment seems to be a stronger protective factor for girls in the development of problems of behaviour at school, whereas for boys this is the case for a positive classroom environment. This model accounted for 40% of the variance in aggression at school for boys and 35% for girls.

Sun et al. (2008) explore family communication patterns, types and the correlation between coping style, family communication and well-being among 1,135 university students in Henan. The results of the study revealed significant difference in family communication patterns between male and female students with different parental education levels or students from different types of universities. The university student's family communication pattern was significantly associated with their coping styles and well-being. Accompany significant difference in family communication pattern shifting, coping style and well-being of university students.

Usha and Lakshmi (2008) studied the influence of parenting style and self-compression on secondary school student's mental health. Sample of the study consisted of 500 students from six schools of Pathanamthitta and three schools of Alappuzha district of Kerala state. The findings of the study indicate that, the main effect of parenting style on mental health was found to be significant for aided school students and non-significant for students of government schools. In the same way the main effect of self-compassion was found to be significant on mental health for the total sample and the subject samples based on the type of school management, sex and locale. The interaction effect of self-compassion and parenting style on mental health was found to be significant for the total sample and subject samples based on locale, type of school management and sex.

Babak et al. (2007) investigated the relationships between general self-efficacy, perceived stress and mental health status among Iranian male adolescents taken from Tehran who studied in senior secondary school. The findings of the study revealed that greater level of stress was associated with lower mental health status and lower general self-efficacy. The results of the study also showed a significant inverse relationship between self-efficacy and general health status of the students.

Carneiro et al. (2007) studied the intergenerational effects of maternal education on children's cognitive achievement, behavioral problems, grade repetition and obesity. Results showed substantial intergenerational returns to education. For children aged 7-8, for example, their IV results indicated that an additional year of mother's schooling increases the child's performance on a standardized math test by almost 0.1 of a standard deviation, and reduced the incidence of behavioral problems. They found that income effects, delayed childbearing, and assortative mating are likely to be important, and they showed that maternal education leads to substantial differences in maternal labor supply. They investigated heterogeneity in returns, and presented results focusing both on very early stages in the child's life as well as adolescent outcomes. They presented a falsification exercise to support the validity of their instruments, and their results were found to be robust in a sensitivity analysis.

Chris et al. (2007) studied social skills, psychological well-being and the mediating role of perceived stress in a sample of 500 university students. The results of the study revealed a significant relationship between social skills and lower levels of perceived stress as well as social skills and greater well-being. The lower levels of perception of stress that accompany higher levels of social skills mediate the association between social skills and depression as well as life satisfaction of students.

Marsiglia et al. (2007) examined the impact of Locus of Control (LOC) and Perceptions of parenting Styles (PS) on the Psycho Social Success (PSS) of Emerging Adults (EAs). PSS was defined as the successful resolution of the tasks postulated by Erikson's stage theory of psychosocial development (1975). The Measures of Psychosocial Development (based on Erikson's theory; Hawley 1988), the Parental Authority Questionnaire (Buri 1991), and the Internal-External scale of Rotter (1966) were completed by 334 undergraduates (ages 18-25). Analyses revealed associations between (1) authoritative parenting and PSS, (2) maternal authoritative parenting and internal LOC, and (3) external LOC and maternal permissive and authoritarian PS. The relation between paternal PS and PSS was also moderated by LOC. Emerging adults' PSS might be affected both directly by their perceptions of the PS they encountered earlier in life and indirectly through LOC, which might also be influenced by perceived PS.

Dwairy et al. (2006) studied parenting styles, individuation and mental health in a sample of 2,893 adolescents retrieved from Arab societies. The results of the study indicated that within an authoritarian culture authoritarian parenting does not harm the adolescent's mental health condition, as it does within the western Liberal societies.

Gibson and Jefferson (2006) examine the effect of perceived parental involvement and the use of growth fostering relationship of self-concept among 78 adolescents who were participated in GEAR-UP (Gaining Early Awareness of Readiness for Undergraduate Programs). The results of the study supported the influence of peers, mentors, family and involvement in community groups on adolescent's self-concept.

Yu et al. (2004) explore the statistical differences existing in well-being of public and private college students also to investigate the interaction among self-concept, well-being and life events of 604 public and private college students. The results of the study obtained demonstrated as follows: (1) self-concept and well-being of private college students were significantly lower than that of public ones, (2) well-being of public and private college students apparently associated with self-concept, whereas negatively correlated with students negative life events, (3) well-being of public college students was mainly affected by identity and personal self (4) well-being of private college students was greatly affected by social self and personal self.

Ciarrochi et al. (2003) explores the relation between social and emotional competence and mental health among 331 university students. They studied stressful life events and a wide variety of social emotional competence measures including alexithymia (describing emotions minimizing emotions and difficulty identity), social problem solving skills (effective problem orientation, automatic processing and problem solving), level of emotional awareness and effective emotional control (high impulse control, low rumination, low defensive inhibiting of emotions and high aggressive control) including wide variety of different aspects of social and mental health (hopelessness, depression, anxiety, suicidal ideation, social support and life satisfaction) of students. The findings of the study revealed that except minimizing the emotions all social emotional competence measures in predicting social competence and mental health of students.

Linares et al. (2002) examined the relationship between parenting styles and 372 adolescents' (aged 11-15 years) psychosocial competence. Parents were classified according to the adolescent's perception in 4 groups: permissive, authoritative, authoritarian and neglectful. Several aspects related to the adolescents' psychosocial competence were assessed through self-report measures. Results showed that both adolescents perceiving their parents as permissive and adolescents perceiving their parents as authoritative obtained the highest scores in perceived social competence and self-esteem. Moreover, their behavior in the classroom was more positive, and they were less rejected by their classmates these findings were discussed in terms of the dimensions of acceptance and control underlying the various parenting styles.

Shek (2002) conducted study to examine the association between family functioning and adjustment in 1,519 Chinese adolescents using an indigenously developed measure of family functioning. Results showed that family functioning was significantly associated with measures of adolescent's school adjustment (satisfaction with academic performance, school conduct and perceived academic performance), problem behaviour (substance abuse and delinquent behavior) and psychological well-being (life satisfaction, existential well-being, self-esteem, general psychiatric morbidity and sense of mastery). Further findings also showed that family functioning was generally more strongly correlated to measures of adjustment for adolescents with economic disadvantage than for adolescents without economic disadvantage.

Aunola et al. (2000) investigates the extent to which adolescent's achievement strategies associated with the parenting styles adolescents experience with their families. The sample of the study consists of 354 adolescents. Results showed that adolescents from authoritative families applied most adaptive achievement strategies characterized by low levels of task irrelevant behaviour, passivity, failure expectations and the use of self-enhancing attributions. However, adolescents from neglectful families in turn applied maladaptive strategies characterized by a lack of self-enhancing attributions and high level of task irrelevant behaviour including passivity.

Medvedova and Luba (2000) investigated the relationship between family environment, parental behaviour and self-esteem in a sample of 391 early adolescents. The results of the study show that in all subjects there was a positive relationship of self-esteem with organization, cohesion, expressiveness and recreational orientation in a family environment. In addition male adolescents self-esteem was positively related to moral global opinion orientation and negatively with cultural family orientation, also highly significant relationship were found between self-esteem and family conflict in all adolescent subjects. Moreover subjects from high conflict families had a lower level of self-esteem, higher anxiety and weaker inward control.

Discussion on Stated Reviews

The above mentioned reviews on home environment and personality variables affecting the mental health of adolescent girls states that parental care was associated with high self-confidence while parental pressure associated with high anxiety. Disturbed families contributed to adolescent anxiety, inability to share personal problems, parental interference in personal affairs and academic pressure. Parental traits were found to negatively influence mental health, e.g., anxiety, adjustment, self-concept and self-confidence. Findings suggest a need for expanding school guidance and counseling capacity to assist parents and adolescents with developmental tasks. Findings also showed that family functioning was generally more strongly correlated to measures of adjustment for adolescents with economic disadvantage than for adolescents without economic disadvantage. Adolescents from neglectful families in turn applied maladaptive strategies characterized by a lack of self-enhancing attributions and high level of task irrelevant behaviour including passivity. The results of the study show that in all subjects there was a positive relationship of self-esteem with organization, cohesion, expressiveness and recreational orientation in a family environment. Significant relationship were found between self-esteem and family conflict in all adolescent subjects.

Conclusion

The review of literature and related studies is very important because such reviewed literature and studies serve as a foundation of the proposed study. This is because related literature and studies guide the researcher in pursuing the research venture. It facilitates a cohesive and integrated approach to the problems and serves a number of important functions in the research process. A crucial element of all research degrees is the review of relevant literature. So important is this chapter that its omission represents a void or absence of a major element in research.

CHAPTER III

RESEARCH METHODOLOGY

Introduction

Research is systematic and organized effort to investigate a specific problem that needs a solution. It contributes to the general body of knowledge. It also corrects human knowledge. Social research now can be defined as the systematic and objective analysis and recording of controlled observations that may lead to the development of generalization, principles or theories resulting in prediction and possibly ultimate control of events in society. It attempts to answer or solve social problems.

According to P.V. Young: "Social research is a scientific undertaking which by means of logical methods, aim to discover new acts or old facts and to analyze their sequences, interrelationships, casual explanations and natural laws which govern them." The Advanced Learner's Dictionary of Current English lays down the meaning of research as "a careful investigation or inquiry especially through search for new facts in any branch of knowledge." Research is an academic activity and as such the term should be used in a technical sense.

Social Work Research

Social work research is the application of research methods to solve problems that social workers confront in the practice of social work. It provides information that can be taken into consideration by social workers prior to making decisions that affect their clients, programmes or agencies such as use of alternative intervention techniques or change or modification of programme/client/objectives and so forth. The designing of research problems, data collection and its interpretation will have to be attempted in a manner as would be useful to professional social work which would add new knowledge to the social work theory and practice and improve the efficiency of professional social workers.

Social work research process is regarded as the systematic use of research concepts, methods, techniques and strategies to provide information related to the objectives of social work programmes and practices. Thus the unit of analysis of social work research could be individuals, groups, families or programme of the agency. That is, social work research, typically focuses on assessment of practitioner's work with individuals, groups, families, communities or appraisal Social Work Intervention with Communities and Institutions of agencies or programmes that involve the continued efforts of practitioners with many clients. As such, the research design, data collection and analytic strategies in social work research vary as a function of unit of analysis and programme of agencies of social work practitioner.

Social work research is the use of the scientific method in the search of knowledge, including knowledge of alternate practice and intervention techniques, which would be of direct use to the social work profession and thus enhance the practice of social work methods. Under social work research, varieties of evaluative researches are undertaken. Some of the researches are on impacts or effects, efficacy and effectiveness. Evaluation of agencies and its projects and programmes are some of the specialized areas of social work research.

Research is, thus, an original contribution to the existing stock of knowledge making for its advancement. It is the pursuit of truth with the help of study, observation, comparison and experiment.

Research Methodology

Research methodology is a way to systematically solve the research problem. It may be understood as a science of studying how research is done scientifically. In this we study the various steps that are generally adopted by a researcher in studying his research problem along with the logic behind them. It is necessary for the researcher to know not only the research methods/techniques but also the methodology. Researchers also need to understand the assumptions underlying various techniques and they need to know the criteria by which they can decide that certain techniques and procedures will be applicable to certain problems and others will not. All this means that it is necessary for the researcher to design his methodology for his problem as the same may differ from problem to problem.

Methodology is defined "as the study of methods by which we gain knowledge. It deals with the cognitive processes imposed on research by the problems arising from the nature of its subject-matter. “Methodology thus prepares the investigator to adopt techniques to neutralize the effects of such hurdles. Research methodology is the description, explanation and justification of various methods of conducting research.

The search for knowledge through objective and systematic method of finding solution to a problem is research. The systematic approach concerning generalization and the formulation of a theory is also research. As such the term ‘research’ refers to the systematic method consisting of enunciating the problem, formulating a hypothesis, collecting the facts or data, analyzing the facts and reaching certain conclusions either in the form of solutions towards the concerned problem or in certain generalizations for some theoretical formulation.

Methodology, does not describe specific methods despite the attention given to the nature and kinds of processes to be followed in a given procedure or in attaining an objective. When proper to a study of methodology, such processes constitute a constructive generic framework; thus they may be broken down in sub-processes, combined, or their sequence changed. As such, methodology may entail a description of generic processor, metaphorically, may be extended to explications of philosophically coherent concepts or theories as they relate to a particular discipline or field of inquiry. By similar reasoning methodology refers to the rationale and the philosophical assumptions that underlie a particular study or a particular methodology.

Statement of the Problem

Adolescence is a period of not only development but also adjustment. During this period the girls get awareness of pressures on them and the necessary relationships. They even develop decision making ability. They want to build personal relationships with someone with whom they can share their hopes and fears, joys and sorrows and their secrets.

According to World Health Organization (WHO) Mental Health includes "Subjective well-being, perceived self-efficacy, autonomy, competence, intergenerational dependence, and self-actualization of one's intellectual and emotional potential, among others." WHO further states that the well-being of an individual is encompassed in the realization of their abilities, coping with normal stresses of life, productive work and contribution to their community. However, cultural differences, subjective assessments, and competing professional theories all affect how "mental health" is defined. A person struggling with his or her behavioral health may face stress, depression, anxiety, relationship problems, grief, addiction, ADHD or learning disabilities, mood disorders, or other psychological concerns. Counselors, therapists, life coaches, psychologists, nurse practitioners or physicians can help manage behavioral health concerns with treatments such as therapy, counseling, or medication. The new field of global mental health is "the area of study, research and practice that places a priority on improving mental health and achieving equity in mental health for all people worldwide". Some mental health clinics are now identified by the phrase behavioral wellness.

Evidence from the World Health Organization suggests that nearly half of the world's population is affected by mental illness with an impact on their self-esteem, relationships and ability to function in everyday life. An individual's emotional health can also impact physical health and poor mental health can lead to problems such as substance abuse. Maintaining good mental health is crucial to living a long and healthy life. Good mental health can enhance one's life, while poor mental health can prevent someone from living an enriching life. Behaviors could be direct reflection of their mental health. Self-destructive acts may take place to suppress emotions. Some of these acts include drug and alcohol abuse, physical fights or vandalism.

Adolescents and Mental Health

Many mental health problems emerge in middle adolescence. Poor mental health can have effect on the wider health and development of adolescents and is associated with several health and social outcomes such as higher alcohol, tobacco and illicit substances use, adolescent pregnancy, unwanted abortions, consequences of abortions, school dropout and delinquent behaviours. There is growing consensus that healthy development during childhood and adolescence contributes to good mental health and can prevent mental health problems. Enhancing social skills, problem-solving skills and self-confidence can help prevent mental health problems such as conduct disorders, anxiety, depression and eating disorders as well as other risk behaviors including those that relate to sexual behavior, substance abuse, and violent behaviour. Health workers need to have the competencies to relate to young people, to detect mental health problems early, and to provide treatments which include counseling, cognitive-behavioral therapy and, where appropriate, psychotropic medication.

Aim

The aim of the present study is to analyze the impact of personality and home environment factors and its influence on mental health of adolescent girls.

Objectives of the Study

1. To assess the mental health status of adolescent girls.
2. To study and find out whether mental health issues give rise to physical and psychological disturbances.
3. To determine the factors affecting mental health and to find out its intensity on adolescent girls.
4. To understand the dimensions of personality of adolescent girls affecting their mental health.
5. To assess the influence of home environment and mental health of the respondents.
6. To understand coping strategies adopted by adolescent girls in dealing with psychological disturbances
7. To offer suggestions from the perspectives of intervention among adolescents.

Hypotheses

To Kerlinger (1968) "Hypothesis is the most powerful tool man has invented to achieve dependable knowledge" (p. 27). It is a powerful tool for the advancement of knowledge because it serves as the working instrument or the tentacles of theory and a means for seeking solution to human problems. Hypotheses are derivable from theory and they serve as means through which theories are validated, revised or invalidated through research (Glassman, 2007). The researcher had formulated some null hypotheses.

They are as follows:

1. There is no significant difference in the Mental Health and Home Environment of the adolescent girls.
2. There is no significant difference in the Home environment and mental health of students.
3. There is no significant difference in the personality traits and mental health of the adolescent girls
4. There is a significant difference in the educational qualification of the father and mental health of their wards.
5. There is a no significant difference in the mental health of students based on their age.
6. There is no significant difference in the mental health of students based on their birth order.
7. There is no significant difference in the mental health of students based on the monthly family income.
8. There is no significant difference in the opinion of students on home environment based on their age.
9. There is no significant difference in the opinion of students on home environment based on father's education.
10. There is no significant difference in the opinion on home environment of students based on the number of members at home.

Title of the Study

The title of the study is, Mental Health of Adolescent Girls.

Research Design

A research design is a logical and systematic plan prepared for directing a research plan. It specifies the objectives of the study, the methodology and techniques to be adopted for achieving the objectives. It constitutes the blue print for the collection, measurement and analysis of data. Research design is needed because it facilitates the smooth sailing of the various research operations thereby making research as efficient as possible yielding maximal information and minimal expenditure of effort, time and money.

The researcher had used descriptive research design in the study as the study is used to describe the factors of mental health and its influence on adolescent girls inspecting on their personality traits and their home environment. Descriptive research studies are those studies which are concerned with describing the characteristics of a particular individual or a group. Those studies concerned with specific predictions with narration of fact that characteristics concerning individual groups or situations are example of descriptive research. The descriptive survey method is used in the present investigation. It describes the current position of the research work. It involves interpretation, comparison, measurement, classification, evaluation and generalization. All these direct towards a proper understanding solution of significant adolescent issues. This study describes the mental health of adolescents in the light of Personality and Home environment .It is conducted among plus two students who are studying in girls higher secondary schools of Palakkad district.

This chapter includes main sections like; design of the study and descriptions of tools. "A research design is the arrangement of conditions for collection and analysis of data in a manner that aims to combine relevance to the research purpose with economy in procedure." In fact, the research design is the conceptual structure within which research is conducted; it constitutes the blueprint for the collection, measurement and analysis of data. Research design stands for advance planning of the methods to be adopted for collecting the relevant data and the techniques to be used for their analysis keeping in view of the research objectives. Design of the study is an essential part of a research project, because design provides a picture of what and how to do the work before starting. It has been determined from time to time that a suitable research design guards against the collection of irrelevant data and grate more economy. So in any research project, design provides the researcher a blueprint of research which dictates the boundaries of project and helps in controlling the experimental, extraneous error, variances of the problem under investigation etc.

This is a correlation study. It correlates mental health with home environment and personality of adolescent girls. The present chapter describes the design or plan of the study and highlights the details about the research procedure followed in conducting the study. As such, it is an important part of the research study and needs to be planned and carried out systematically to arrive at accurate judgements. It includes information about the population, the sample frame, the nature and form of data collection, tools, methods of collecting data and statistical techniques used for analysis of data etc. In order to achieve the objectives and the stated corresponding hypotheses the following plan of the study has been followed. Method of research is also determined by the theory and objectives of the problem to be studied. The problem to be investigated for the present study concerns with adolescent girls in higher secondary schools in relation to their home environment, personality and mental health.

Pilot Study

Pilot study is a cardinal role in research that one must 'try out' or pilot test the questionnaire to find out whether it operates properly before using it in a research study. The following are some of objectives of a pilot study. A pilot study was conducted by the researcher as a preliminary step to get familiar with the topic. The researcher made a questionnaire with necessary details and interviewed some respondents to start the study. The researcher conducted the pilot study:

1) To examine the scope of the study.
2) To see whether necessary information can be collected.
3) To determine the method and tools of data collection.
4) To find out the availability of data.
5) To fix universe of the study.
6) To select the sampling design.
7) To identify weak and defective items.
8) To find out the discriminating power of each item.

9) To provide data needed to determine how many items should constitute the final form of the tool.

10) To decide the proper format.

Through the pilot study the investigator found out that there is ample scope for the study as the topic is relevant and also growing issue from every perspective.

Construction of the Questionnaire

The researcher referred various books, magazines and journals in order to understand various aspects of mental health of adolescent girls. Literature review enabled the researcher to gather more information regarding the adolescent and their various issues. The researcher was able to prepare the questionnaire on the basis of the literature survey.

Pre – Test

A pretest was carried out with Thirty - six respondents before carrying out the study. Certain modifications were made in the questionnaire after the pre – test and the modified questionnaire was used for the present study. It was conducted to test the effectiveness, relevance and applicability of the questions in the context.

Universe and Sampling

The universe of the research that the researcher had chosen for the study were all girl students studying in plus two classes in different schools in Palakkad city. Total number of higher secondary schools in Palakkad city is 25 comprising of government, special, un-aided aided minority, aided general and aided backward schools. Among the total 25 schools only 6 schools are not offering co-education and are girls schools, those school students is the population of the present study. Population of the study is 1440. The sample size of the study is fixed to 360. Robert V. Krejcie and Daryle W. Morgan (1970) gave a population sample-size guideline based on its calculated representation of its population. They have suggested that size of sample for population of 1400-1500 can be fixed between 302-306. To minimize chances of a sampling error, researcher decided to increase sample size to 360 (Table 1).

Sampling Design

Sampling design refers to the technique which is used for selection of the items for the sample in a research Probability sampling is used in the study. Probability sampling is the method of sampling that utilizes some form of random selection which assures that different units in the population have equal probabilities of being chosen.. Stratified random sampling is used in the present study. Stratified random sampling is a probability sampling technique, it is also known as proportional random sampling. This is a probability sampling technique wherein the subjects are initially grouped into different classifications such as age group of 15-17 years, income of the family, ownership of the school. Then, the researcher randomly finds out the final list of subjects from the different strata. It is important to note that all the strata must have no overlaps.

Researchers also employ stratified random sampling when they want to observe existing relationships between two or more subgroups. With a simple random sampling technique, the researcher is not sure whether the subgroups that he wants to observe are represented equally or proportionately within the sample. With stratified sampling, the researcher can representatively sample even the smallest and most inaccessible subgroups in the population. This allows the researcher to sample the rare extremes of the given population. With this technique, you have a higher statistical precision compared to simple random sampling. This is because the variability within the subgroups is lower compared to the variations when dealing with the entire population.

Because this technique has high statistical precision, it also means that it requires a small sample size which can save a lot of time, money and effort of the researchers. Researchers usually use stratified random sampling if they want to study a particular subgroup within the population. Within the strata, the researcher have used the lottery method for the purpose of finding out the samples for the study. It is also preferred over the simple random sampling because it warrants more precise statistical outcomes.

Table 1

Table Depicting the Samples

Sl. No	Name of the school	School Strength	Strength of plus two girls	Sample break up
1	Govt. Moyan Model Girls HSS, Palakkad	232	116	58
2	Govt. Girls HSS Alathur, Palakkad	236	118	59
3	Cherupushpam Girls HSS, Palakkad	240	120	60
4	St.Therese HSS Shornur, Palakkad	244	122	61
5	Govt. Girls HSS, Nemmara, Palakkad	236	118	59
6	LSN Girls HSS Ottapalam, Palakkad	252	126	63
	Total	**1440**	**720**	**360**

Tools of Data Collection

The researcher had adopted questionnaire method for the purpose of collecting data from the respondents. It was used to find out the mental health of adolescent girls in relation to their home environment and personality traits. The questionnaire consists of 4 parts. First part consists of personal profile and the second part consists of mental health inventory which consists of questions relating to mental health dimensions and it is 55 questions together.

Mental Health Inventory (MHI) (Jagdish & Srivastav, 1983)

Mental health inventory (MHI) developed by Jagdish and Srivastav (1983) was utilized to access positive aspects of mental health. This test can be used as a group or an individual test, for ages 15 and above, no time and age limit is enforced in the testing. Each items from 1 to 56 given in the test booklet to be rated on 4 point rating scale. It covers the following 6 dimensions of sound mental health

(1) Positive Self-Evaluation (PSE) – self-confidence, self-acceptance, self-identity, realization of one's capabilities.

(2) Perception of Reality (PR) – related to absence of excessive fantasy, ability to face and accept realities of life.

(3) Integration of Personality (IP) – indicates balance of psychological forces in the individual, includes emotional maturity, ability to concentrate at work and interest in several activities.

(4) Autonomy (AUT) – the actions of people are independent rater than dependant on other persons.

(5) Group Oriented Attitudes (GOA) – ability to work with others and ability to find recreation.

(6) Environment Mastery

(EM) – Efficiency in meeting situational demands.

Reliability of the Inventory

The reliability of the inventory was determined by 'split half' methods using odd even procedure (Table 2)

Table 2

Table Presenting Reliability Co-efficient

Sl. No.	Dimensions of M.H.	Reliability Index
1	Positive self evaluation	.75
2	Perception of reality	.71
3	Integration of personality	.72
4	Autonomy	.72
5	Group oriented attitude	.74
6	Environment competence	.71
	Overall evaluation	.73

Construct validity of the inventory is determined by finding coefficient of correction between scores on mental health inventory and general health questionnaire (gold berg, 1978) it was found to be 54 it is note worthy here that high score on the general questionnaire indicates poor mental health. Two inventory scores yield positive correlation of (.57) revealing moderate validity. The test is scored with the help of manual. 4 alternative responses have been given to each statement i.e. always often, rarely ad never. 4 scores to always, 3 scores to often, 2 scores to rarely and 1 scores to never, marked responses are to be assigned for true keyed (positive) statements where as 1, 2, 3 and 4 scores for always, 'often' rarely and never respectively in case of false keyed (negative) statements.

Personality Inventory Scale (B.L. Dubey, P. Dwivedi and S. K. Verma, 1988)

The Personality Inventory was constructed and standardized by B.L. Dubey, P. Dwivedi and S. K. Verma in 1988 and was used in this study. The Inventory consists of 50 statements. The Personality Inventory Scale is used to measure certain well known dimensions of personalities like

a. Extraversion

b. Psychotism

c. Emotional instability

d. Depression

e. Social Desirability

Among the 50 statements, the Extraversion statements are (No.) 9, 14, 19, 24, 34, 39, 44, 49.

Psychotism statements are (No.) 1, 3, 6, 8, 11, 13 16, 17, 21, 28, 31, 33, 43, 48, 36, 37, 38, 41.

Emotional instability statements are (No.) 4, 20, 23, 40, 42.

Depression statements are (No.) 2, 7, 12, 18, 22, 27, 32, 46, 47.

Social Desirability statements are (No.) 5, 10, 15, 25, 26, 29, 30, 35, 45, 50. The reliability of this scale is 0.682.

The third part consists of personality inventory for the assessment of personality traits of adolescent girls and it consists of 50 questions and the fourth part consists of home environment inventory developed by Dr. SarlaJawa is adopted in this study. This scale is of Likert type and has items related to personal freedom, rapport with parents and siblings, interpersonal relations, for understanding the influence of home atmosphere on the mental health of girls and it is 22 questions in number, in final version after the modifications.

The variables used in the study are independent variables and dependent variables. The various independent variables are age, class, educational qualification of parents, birth order, family income, size of the family and the number of siblings.

The various dependent variables used in the study are the home environment factors, Personality factors and also dimensions like decision making skill, confidence level, reality orientation, loneliness, rejection etc.

Analysis of Data

The analysis of the data is the most skilled task in the research process. It calls for the researchers own judgment and skill. Analysis of data involves the re-categorization of variables, tabulation, explanation and casual inference. One way tables or frequency tables and two way tables or cross tables were used for the purpose of analysis. The collected data were entered to a master sheet to make tabulation and analysis easier.

Analysis is the vital part of the study, because the findings, suggestions and conclusions of the study are mainly based on the analysis. The statistical tools applied in the present study were Mean, Standard Deviation, Chi-Square, t test, One Way Anova, Co-relation, Regression and Factor Analysis.

This provided the investigator with the data which is presented in the next chapter. The analysis and interpretation of this data is also demonstrated in the following chapters.

Scope of the Study

The present research tries to bring out the relationship of mental health and its influence on home environment and personality factors of higher secondary girl students. But any study, however, wide it may be, its scope cannot claim to be all inclusive and points out the scope for further investigation with other equally relevant variables. In an attempt for solution of the problem, new problems arise. It is from this point of view, some suggestions are being made for further investigation of some of the important issues that seem to originate from the present work.

1. The study can also be conducted with the sample of primary and senior secondary school students.
2. The study can also be undertaken to find the relationship and significance of difference among other cognitive and non-cognitive attributes.
3. Similar studies may also be taken to study the variables like socio-economic status, rural and urban etc.
4. A similar study can be conducted on a group of arts and science students.
5. A study of special group of students may be undertaken.
6. Comparative study can be conducted with reference to creative students and with different level of intelligence.

Problems faced by the Researcher

- Some respondents were absent on the day of returning the questionnaire.
- The researchers have to assure the respondents to maintain confidentiality as they were curious, shy and fearful.
- Some respondents were less interested in the research and hence some refused first to return back the questionnaire.
- At times the researcher also lost certain questionnaire as some of them were having incomplete information.

Limitations of the Study

- It is a time bound study.
- As the study has been done among small population, the finding cannot be generalized.
- The study only limited to girls schools and hence generalization on both genders cannot be made.
- This study is limited only to schools within Palakkad city, hence the result cannot be applied to all the schools in entire Palakkad district.

Operational Definitions of the Concept

Adolescent: Adolescent girls are those who are in the age group between 15 to 17 years of age of girl's higher secondary schools in Palakkad. For the purpose of this study a girl student studying in class XII in any recognized or private school is considered as adolescent.

Mental Health: Mental health of adolescents were assessed by covering six main dimensions like positive self-evaluation, realistic perception, integrity of personality, autonomy, group oriented activity, environmental mastery.

Personality: Personality is the particular combination of cognitive, emotional, attitudinal, and behavioral response patterns of an individual reflecting in the following dimensions-extraversion, emotional instability, depression, social desirability, dimensions of personality, Competition, enthusiasm, innovation, leadership, maturity, mental health, morality, self-control, sensitivity, self-sufficiency, and social warmth.

Nature of the home environment: The encouragement, discouragement, understanding or negligence, imposition, scope for expression of one's interests and wishes at home influence the development of child's personality. Various areas of focus includes social isolation, personal freedom, Rapport with parents and siblings, interparental relations. Hence the nature of home environment is taken as a variable for study.

Chapterization

The thesis has been organized in the following way:

The **first chapter** deals with the Introduction of the study, its related concepts, and objectives of the study, need and significance of the study.

The **second chapter** deals with the Review of Literature.

The **third chapter** consists of the Introduction, statement of the problem, title of the study, research design, pilot study, construction of the questionnaire, pre-test, universe of the study sampling design, tools of data collection, statistical analysis of data, scope of the study, problems faced by the researcher, limitations of the study and the operational definitions.

The **fourth chapter** deals with the Analysis and Interpretation of the collected data.

The **fifth chapter** deals with Findings, Suggestions and Conclusions.

This is followed by Bibliography and Annexure.

Conclusion

Research Methodology is a systematic way to solve the research problem. Social work research focuses on or confines itself to select aspects of behaviour and alternate models of behaviour modifications. Social work research helps to find ways and means to enhance social functioning at the individual, group, community and societal levels. Social work research lays special emphasis on evaluation. This is one of the reasons that social work research is also understood as evaluative research. The procedures by which researchers go about their work of describing, explaining and predicting phenomena are called methodology. All the methods used by social scientists in their fact-finding mission constitute methodology. Research Methodology has many dimensions and research methodology constitute a part of the research. This whole chapter is engaged in employing research methodology which consist of certain scientific steps for successful execution and objectively. In this chapter the research design and sampling technique was given in detail. The procedure for construction and finalization of the tool was also described. The collected questionnaires were scored properly and suitable statistical analysis was carried out. The details of analysis and discussion are given in the next chapter.

CHAPTER IV

ANALYSIS AND INTERPRETATION

Introduction

The researcher had discussed in chapter three, the research design and methodology, origin of the research, design of the research, variable of the research, population and sample of the research, tools for data collection, procedure for data collection, statistical analysis done in research work. Data analysis is consider to be important step and heart of the research in research work. After collection of data with the help of relevant tools and techniques, the next logical step, is to analyze and interpret data with a view to arriving at empirical solution to the problem. The data analysis for the present research was done quantitatively with the help of both descriptive statistics and inferential statistics.

Table 3

Distribution of Respondents by their Personal Details

Particulars		No	Percent
Medium of instruction	English	160	44.4
	Malayalam	200	55.6
Age	15	20	5.6
	16	240	66.7
	17	100	27.8
Birthorder	First	130	36.1
	Second	120	33.3
	Third	80	22.2
	Fourth	30	8.3
Father's education	Primary	60	16.7
	Secondary	260	72.2
	Higher Secondary	40	11.1

Particulars		No	Percent
Mother's education	Primary	90	25.0
	Secondary	190	52.8
	Higher Secondary	70	19.4
	Graduate and above	10	2.8
Family Monthly Income	25000 to 50000	30	8.3
	10000 to 25000	40	11.1
	5000 to 10000	130	36.1
	Below 5000	160	44.4
Family size	5 to 10	190	52.8
	Less than 5	160	44.4
	5	10	2.8
Total		**360**	**100.0**

The above table indicates that 44.4 percent of the respondents belong to English medium of instruction. 55.6 percent of the respondents have been from Malayalam medium of instruction. So, the majority of the respondents have studied in Malayalam medium.

The above table shows the distribution by age. The majority (66.7 %) of the sample size belonged to 16 years of age. Group followed by 27.8 percent of 17 years, 5.6 percent were 15 years and above. It clearly indicates that majority of the students are in middle adolescent age.

Birth order column of the table indicates that 36.1 percent of the respondent are first born, 33.3 percent of the respondents ant second born followed by 22.2 percent of the respondent are third born, and 8.3 percent of the respondent are fourth born. It is clearly evident that majority of the respondents are either first born or second born as two children norm is prevalent for the last few decades. The ordinal position is very important in determining the personality and mental health of the adolescents.

Though the study is conducted in higher secondary schools the education of the parent's was also considered and father's education of the respondents were analysed and the result shows that 72.2 percent of the respondents' fathers are secondary educated and followed by 16.7 percent of fathers are primary educated and 11.1 percent of them are higher secondary educated. Fathers education have role in mental health status of children and adolescents as their influence them.

Mother's education of the respondents were analysed and the result shows that 52.8 percent of the respondents' mothers are secondary educated and followed by 25 percent of mothers are primary educated, 19.4 percent of them are higher secondary educated and only 2.8 percent of them are graduates and above. Mothers education have impact on the personality and mental health of adolescents as they are upbringing their children.

Figure 2

Distribution of Respondents by their Age

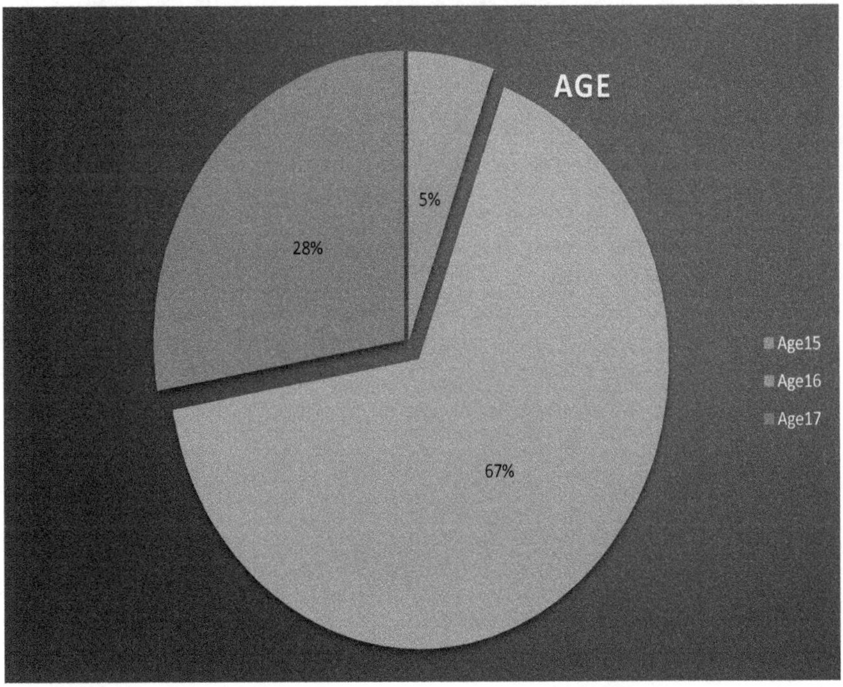

Figure 3

Distribution of Respondents by Birth Order

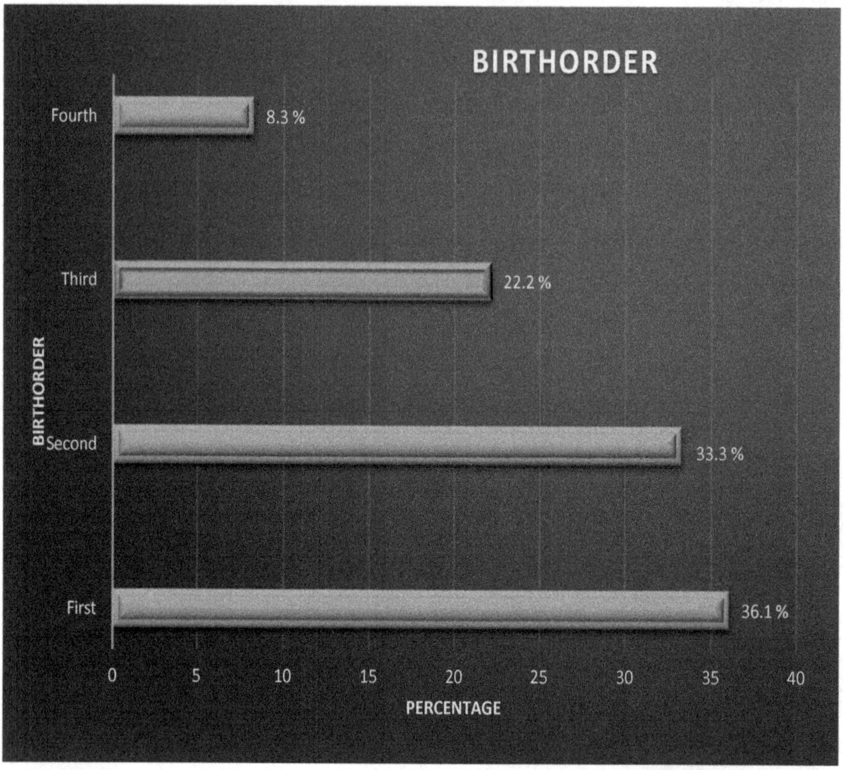

Figure 4

Distribution of Respondents by their Family Monthly Income

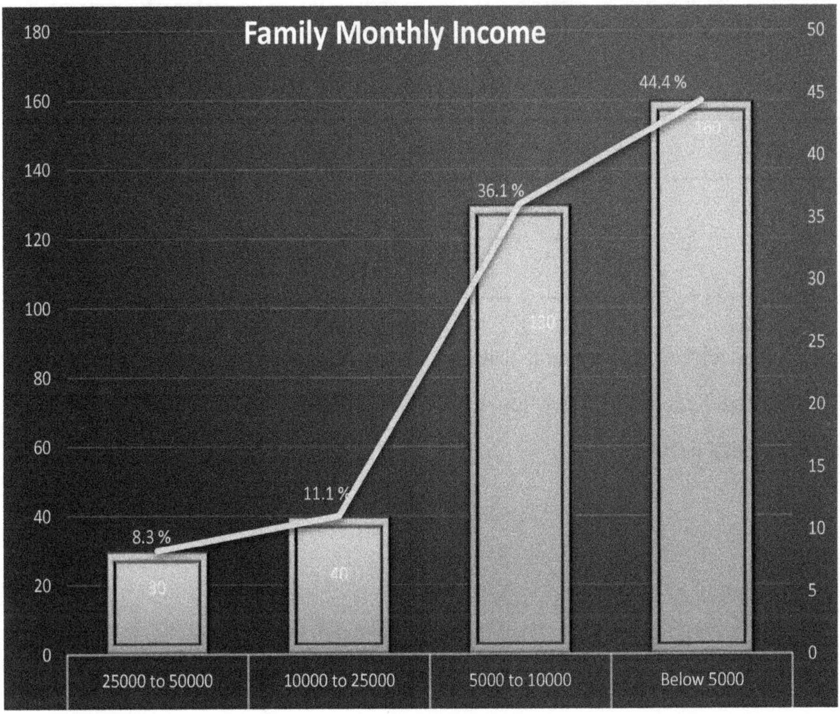

Table 4

Table Demonstrating the Mental Health of the Respondents

Mental health	Frequency	Percent
High	50	13.9
Normal	210	58.3
Low	100	27.8
Total	360	100

It is evident from the table that 13.9% of adolescents have high mental health and 27.8% of adolescent girls have low mental health, but 58.3%of adolescent girls have normal mental health.

Figure 5

Distribution of Respondents by their Mental Health

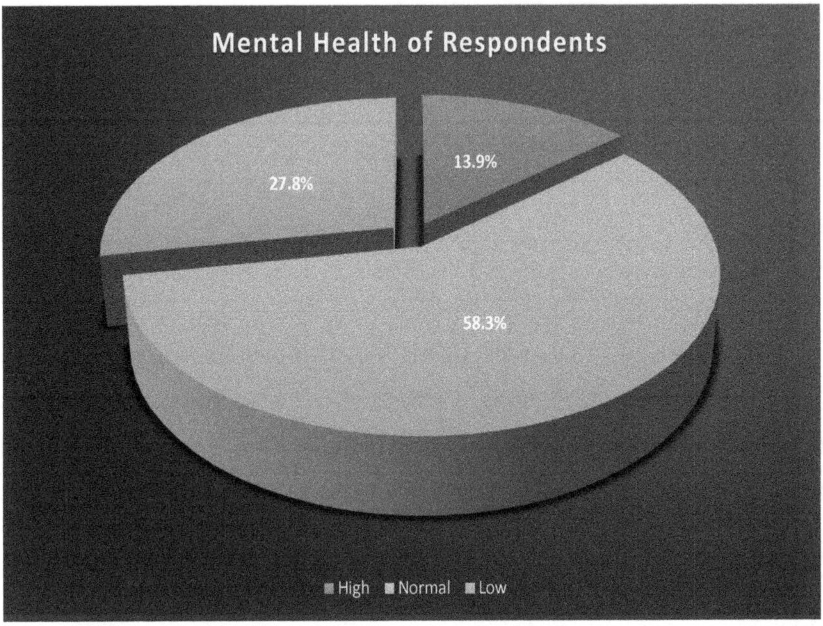

Table 5

Table Showing the Distribution of Respondents by their Home Environment

Home environment	Frequency	Percent
Good	50	13.9
Normal	250	69.4
Poor	60	16.7
Total	360	100

The Adolescent girls learn lot of things from her family. Family plays a major role in her development and behavior formation. The above mentioned states that 69.4 percent of the adolescent girls have normal environment at their home. 16.7 percent of the girls have poor home environment, but the analysis shows that 13.9 percent of them have good environment at their home.

Figure 6

Distribution of Respondents by their Home Environment Condition

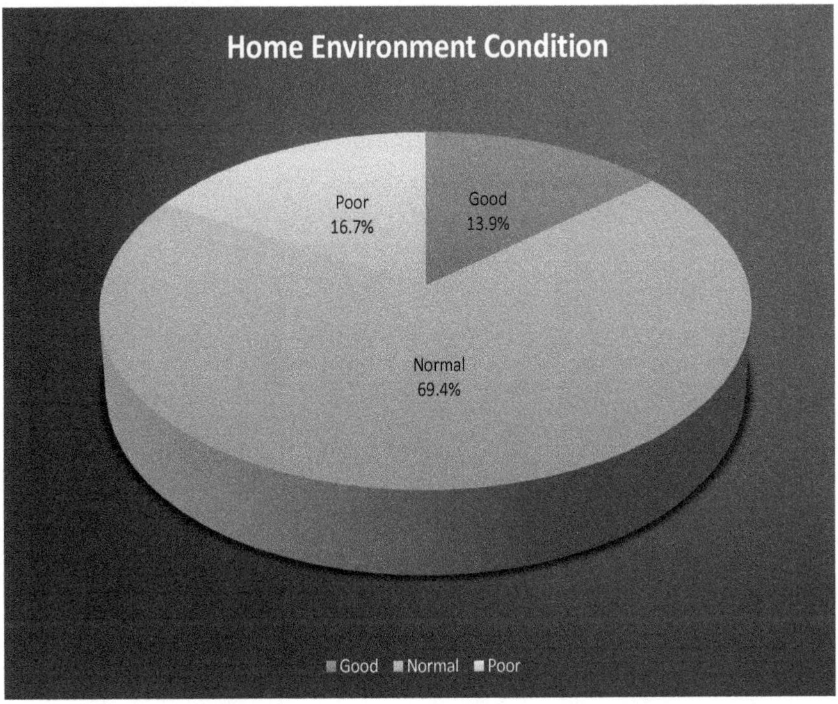

Table 6

Table Indicating Personality Traits of the Adolescent Girls

Personality traits	Frequency	Percent
Low	120	33.3
High	240	66.7
Total	360	100

Personality scores are classified as low and high. The personality inventory scores of the respondents reveals that 66.7 percent of them have high scores in personality and 33.3 percent of them have low scores in personality.

Figure 7

Distribution of Respondents by the Personality Scores of the Adolescent Girls

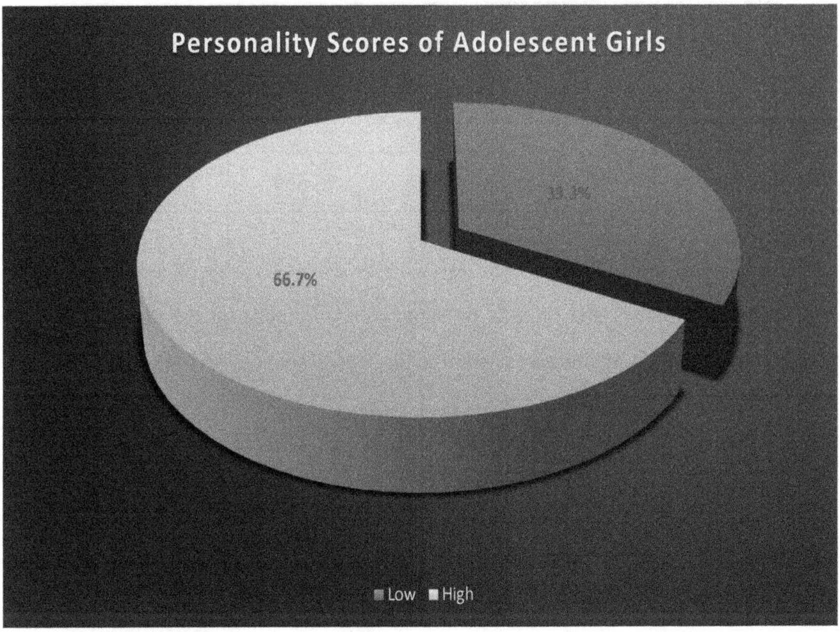

Table 7

Anova Showing Mental Health and Medium of Instruction

	Sum of Squares	df	Mean Square	F	Sig.
Between Groups	62.347	1	62.347	.935	.334
Within Groups	23867.375	358	66.669		
Total	23929.722	359			

The table shows that there is no significant difference on the mental health of students based on their medium instruction as the significant value 0.334 is >0.05

Table 8

Anova Presenting Age and Mental Health

	Sum of Squares	df	Mean Square	F	Sig.
Between Groups	434.139	2	217.069	3.298	.038
Within Groups	23495.583	357	65.814		
Total	23929.722	359			

The table shows that there is a significant difference on the mental health of students based on their age as the significant value (of F = 3.298) 0.038 < 0.05

Age	Mean	N	Std. Deviation
15	136.0000	20	4.10391
16	132.7917	240	8.51275
17	131.2000	100	7.69100
Total	132.5278	360	8.16435

The mean value of the mental health inventory shows that students at the age of 15 have more mental health and the second highest is 16 years old children and it is comparatively low for the students at the age of 17.

Table 9

Anova Indicating Mental Health and Birth Order

	Sum of Squares	df	Mean Square	F	Sig.
Between Groups	124.530	3	41.510	.621	.602
Within Groups	23805.192	356	66.869		
Total	23929.722	359			

It is clear from the above table that there is no significant difference in the mental health of students based on their birth order as the significance value is > 0.05.

Table 10

Anova Depicting Mental Health and Father's Education

	Sum of Squares	**df**	**Mean Square**	**F**	**Sig.**
Between Groups	6105.235	2	3052.618	61.140	.000
Within Groups	17824.487	357	49.929		
Total	23929.722	359			

The above table shows that there is a significant difference in the mental health based on father's education. F= 61.140 is significant at 0.05 level.

Father's Education	**Mean**	**N**	**Std. Deviation**
Primary	123.3333	60	7.97595
Secondary	134.2692	260	7.32351
Higher Secondary	135.0000	40	2.14834
Total	132.5278	360	8.16435

The mean value is high when father's education is more. Hence student's mental health increased when father's education is good.

Table 11

Anova Showing Mental Health and Mother's Education

	Sum of Squares	df	Mean Square	F	Sig.
Between Groups	1364.309	3	454.770	7.175	.000
Within Groups	22565.414	356	63.386		
Total	23929.722	359			

There is a significant difference in the mental health of students based on the mother's education too, as the significant level (of F = 7.175) is < 0.01

Mother's Education	Mean	N	Std. Deviation
Primary	130.3333	90	9.56351
Secondary	132.2632	190	8.67303
Higher Secondary	136.1429	70	1.73861
Graduate and above	132.0000	10	.00000
Total	132.5278	360	8.16435

It is also clear that the mother's education is more the child's mental health also increases except in the case of graduate mother's.

Table 12

Anova Revealing Mental Health and Family Monthly Income

	Sum of Squares	df	Mean Square	F	Sig.
Between Groups	2032.415	3	677.472	11.014	.000
Within Groups	21897.308	356	61.509		
Total	23929.722	359			

There is a significant difference in the mental health of students based on the monthly family income, as the significant level (of $F = 11.014$) is < 0.01

Family Monthly Income	Mean	N	Std. Deviation
25000 to 50000	138.0000	30	4.62378
10000 to 25000	136.2500	40	1.31559
5000 to 10000	132.4615	130	8.73037
Below 5000	130.6250	160	8.45911
Total	132.5278	360	8.16435

The mean value shows that the mental health is more when the income of the increases.

Table 13

Anova for Mental Health and Total Number of Members in the Family

	Sum of Squares	df	Mean Square	F	Sig.
Between Groups	1570.084	2	785.042	12.534	.000
Within Groups	22359.638	357	62.632		
Total	23929.722	359			

There is a significant difference in the mental health of students based on the number of members in the family, as the significant level (of F = 12.534) is < 0.01

Total Members in Family	Mean	N	Std. Deviation
3	132.1579	190	7.62385
4	133.6875	160	8.45795
5	121.0000	10	.00000
Total	132.5278	360	8.16435

The mean value shows that the mental health is more when there are 4 members and it is low when this increases. i.e., students from family of two children father and mother feel better compared to family with grandparents or other relatives and it is also low with students of single child family.

Table 14

Table Showing the Feeling of Respondents on Lack of Confidence

Response	Frequency	Percent
Always	340	94.4
Sometimes	10	2.8
Never	10	2.8
Total	360	100

The above table shows that the respondents feel that 94% of them feel lack of confidence always, but 2.8% of them replied that they feel lack of confidence some times and 2.8% of them opine that they never feel lack of confidence.

Table 15

Table Revealing the Feeling of Respondents on Getting Excited Easily

Response	Frequency	Percent
Always	10	2.8
Most of Times	320	88.9
Sometimes	20	5.6
Never	10	2.8
Total	360	100

The above table shows that the respondents feel that 88.9% of them get excited very easily most of the times, but 5.6% of them replied that they get excited some times, 2.8 %of the feel that they feel excited always and 2.8% of them opine that they never feel easily excited.

Table 16

Table Depicting the Inability of Respondents on Taking Quick Decisions

Response	Frequency	Percent
Always	320	88.9
Most of Times	10	2.8
Sometimes	10	2.8
Never	20	5.6
Total	360	100

The above table indicates that the respondents feel that 88.9% of them believe that they are not able to take quick decision on any subject always, 2.8 % of them feel that they are not able to take quick decision on any subject most of the times, but 2.8 % of them replied that they are not able to take quick decision on any subject some times, and 5.6 % of them opine that they never feel difficulty in taking quick decisions on any subject.

Table 17

Table Presenting the Belief of Respondents that Situations are Continuously Going against them

Response	Frequency	Percent
Always	330	91.7
Most of Times	20	5.6
Sometimes	10	2.8
Total	360	100

The above table shows that 91.7% of the respondents feel that situations are continuously going against them always, 5.6 % of them feel that situations are continuously going against them most of the times, but 2.8 % of them feel that situations are continuously going against them sometimes.

Table 18

Table Showing the Affection and Attachment of the Respondents with their Neighbours

Response	Frequency	Percent
Always	10	2.8
Sometimes	20	5.6
Never	330	91.7
Total	360	100

The above table shows that 91.7% of the respondents feel that they never have affection and attachment with their neighbors, 5.6 % of them feel that they have affection and attachment with their neighbors sometimes, but 2.8 % of them feel that they have affection and attachment with their neighbors always.

Table 19

Table Demonstrating Respondents' Opinion on Adjusting themselves as per Circumstances

Response	Frequency	Percent
Always	10	2.8
Most of Times	10	2.8
Sometimes	110	30.6
Never	230	63.9
Total	360	100.0

The above table indicates that 63.9 % of the respondents opine that they never make adjustments according to the circumstances, 30.6% of them opine that they mould according to circumstances sometimes, 2.8 % of them opine that they make adjustments according to the circumstances most of the times, but only 2.8% of them opine that they make adjustments according to circumstances always.

Table 20

Table Revealing the Belief of the Respondents on Losing Self Respect

Response	Frequency	Percent
Always	100	27.8
Sometimes	250	69.4
Never	10	2.8
Total	360	100

The above table indicates that 69.4 % of the respondents feel that they are losing self respect sometimes, 27.8% of them feel that they are losing self respect always, but 2.8 % of them feel that they never lose self respect.

Table 21

Respondents on Worrying about Trivial Matters for Long Time

Response	Frequency	Percent
Always	10	2.8
Most of Times	100	27.8
Sometimes	230	63.9
Never	20	5.6
Total	360	100

The above table indicates that 63.9 % of the respondents feel that they keep worrying about trivial matters for long time sometimes, 27.8% of them feel that they keep worrying about trivial matters for long time most of the times, 5.6 of them feel that they never keep worrying about trivial matters for long time, but 2.8 % of them feel that they keep worrying about trivial matters for long time always.

Table 22

Table Displaying the Feeling of Hesitation of the Respondents in Meeting Others

Response	Frequency	Percent
Always	350	97.2
Most of Times	10	2.8
Total	360	100

The above table indicates that 97.2% of the respondents feel hesitation in meeting others always and 2.8% of them feel hesitation in meeting others most of the times.

Table 23

Table Showing the Feeling of the Respondents on Doing Duty Well in Adverse Circumstances

Response	Frequency	Percent
Always	40	11.1
Most of Times	100	27.8
Sometimes	200	55.6
Never	20	5.6
Total	360	100

The above table indicates that 55.6% of the respondents feel that they do their duty well even in adverse circumstances sometimes, 27. 8% of them feel that they do their duty well even in adverse circumstances most of the times, 11.1% of them feel that they do their duty well even in adverse circumstances always, but 5.6 % of them feel that they never do their duty well even in adverse circumstances.

Table 24

Classification of Respondents on not able to Fully Utilize their Ability in Performing Duties

Response	Frequency	Percent
Always	120	33.3
Sometimes	150	41.7
Never	90	25.0
Total	360	100

The above table indicates that 41.7% of the respondents feel that they are not able to fully utilize their ability in performing duties sometimes, 33.3% of them feel that they are not able to fully utilize their ability in performing duties always, but 25% of them never feel that they are not able to fully utilize their ability in performing duties.

Table 25

Table Presenting the Feeling of the Respondents in Adverse Circumstances

Response	Frequency	Percent
Always	100	27.8
Most of Times	250	69.4
Sometimes	10	2.8
Total	360	100

The above table shows that 69.4% of the respondents feel that even in adverse circumstances, they act without keeping in view of the real facts most of the times, 27.8% of them feel that even in adverse circumstances, they act without keeping in view of the real facts always, but 2.8% of them feel that even in adverse circumstances, they act without keeping in view of the real facts sometimes.

Table 26

Table Depicting the Feeling of the Respondents on Get Irritated

Response	Frequency	Percent
Always	330	91.7
Most of Times	30	8.3
Total	360	100

The above table shows that 91.7% of the respondents feel that they get irritated always and 8.3% of the respondents feel that they get irritated most of the times.

Table 27

Table Revealing the Opinion of the Respondents on Feeling in Secured

Response	Frequency	Percent
Always	330	91.7
Most of Times	30	8.3
Total	360	100

The above table shows that 91.7% of the respondents opine that they feel insecure always and 8.3% of the respondents feel that they feel insecure most of the times.

Table 28

Table Showing the Opinion of the Respondents on Feeling Worried about Respondents

Response	Frequency	Percent
Always	330	91.7
Most of Times	10	2.8
Sometimes	20	5.6
Total	360	100

The above table shows that 91.7% of the respondents feel that they are much worried about their responsibilities always, 5.6% of them feel that they are much worried about their responsibilities sometimes, but 2.8% of them feel that they are much worried about their responsibilities most of the times.

Table 29

Table Demonstrating the Opinion of Respondents on Feeling Depressed or Dejected

Response	Frequency	Percent
Always	340	94.4
Most of Times	20	5.6
Total	360	100

The above table shows that 94.4% of the respondents opine that they feel depressed or dejected always and 5.6% of the respondents feel that they feel depressed or dejected most of the times.

Discussion

Sally et al. (2012) states that depression is common in young people, has a marked negative impact and is associated with self-harm and suicide. Preventing its onset would be an important advance in public health. To determine whether psychological or educational interventions, or both, are effective in preventing the onset of depressive disorder in children and adolescents. The result is similar to the results of the present study.

Kadison and Digeronimo (2004), in their study have highlighted the campus mental crisis and what to do about it. The paper confirms that a rising number of students are coping with depression anxiety and other major mental health challenges. This finding is contradictory to the results of the present study.

Figure 8

Distribution of Respondents on Feeling Depressed or Dejected

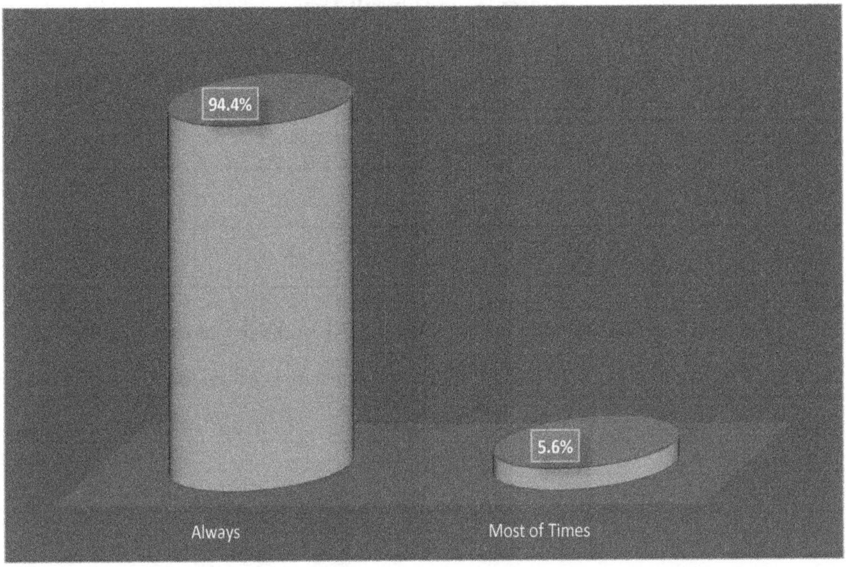

Table 30

Table Exhibiting the Opinion of Respondents on Utilizing Reasoning in Difficult Times

Response	Frequency	Percent
Always	100	27.8
Most of Times	260	72.2
Total	360	100

The above mentioned table indicates that 72.2% of the respondents feel that they are able to utilize their reasoning even in difficult times most of the times and 27.8% of them believe that they are able to utilize their reasoning even in difficult times always.

Table 31

Table Depicting the Feeling of Respondents on Keeping Satisfactory Relations with Others

Response	Frequency	Percent
Always	100	27.8
Most of Times	240	66.7
Sometimes	20	5.6
Total	360	100

The above mentioned table indicates that 66.7% of the respondents feel that their relations with others are not satisfactory most of the times and 27.8% of the respondents feel that their relations with others are not satisfactory always, but 5.6% of them feel that their relations with others are not satisfactory sometimes.

Table 32

Table Presenting the Feeling of Inferiority Complex of the Respondents

Response	Frequency	Percent
Always	320	88.9
Most of Times	40	11.1
Total	360	100

The above mentioned table indicates that 88.9% of the respondents feel inferiority complex always and 11.1% of the respondents feel inferiority complex most of times.

Table 33

Table Indicating the Feeling of to be lost in the World of Imagination by the Respondents

Response	Frequency	Percent
Always	360	100

The above mentioned table indicates that 100.0% of the respondents opined that they feel to be lost in the world of imagination always.

Table 34

Table Exhibiting the Anxiety of the Respondents about their Future

Response	Frequency	Percent
Sometimes	290	80.6
Never	70	19.4
Total	360	100

The table shows that 80.6% of the respondents are anxious about their future sometimes, but 19.4% of the respondents opined that they are never anxious about their future.

Discussion

Levine and Cureton (1998) opines that generally students are coming to educational institutions more damaged and overwhelmed with anxiety than those of previous years. This result is in line with the researcher's present study.

Table 35

Table Demonstrating the Opinion of Respondents on Getting Enraged by the Slightest Unfavorable Task

Response	Frequency	Percent
Most of Times	100	27.8
Sometimes	20	5.6
Never	240	66.7
Total	360	100

The above mentioned table indicates that 66.7% of them opine that they are never enraged by the slightest unfavourable task, 27.8% of the respondents opine that they get enraged by slightest unfavourable task most of the times and 5.6% of the respondents opine that they are enraged even by the slightest unfavorable task sometimes.

Table 36

Table Presenting Belief of the Respondents on their Confidence Level Variation

Response	Frequency	Percent
Sometimes	110	30.6
Never	250	69.4
Total	360	100

The above table indicates that 69.4 % of the respondents believe that their confidence never varies high in quantity, but 30.6% of them believe that their confidence varies high in quantity sometimes.

Table 37

Table Indicating the Willingness of the Respondents to Face and Fight the Problems of Life

Response	Frequency	Percent
Always	30	8.3
Most of Times	200	55.6
Sometimes	130	36.1
Total	360	100

The above mentioned table indicates that 55.6% of the respondents are willing to fight the problems of life most of times, but 36.1% of the respondents are willing to fight the problems of life sometimes, and 8.3% of the respondents are willing to fight the problems of life always.

Discussion

Ashurst et al. (2009) in their study found out that the need to expand the focus in youth development research and practice to include positive developmental outcomes that can result from coping with life crisis during adolescence. This result is similar to the findings of the present study.

Table 38

Table Depicting the Belief of the Respondents on Solving the Problems by their Self

Response	Frequency	Percent
Most of Times	100	27.8
Sometimes	260	72.2
Total	360	100

The above mentioned table indicates that 72.2% of the respondents believe that they can solve their problems by their self most of times, but 27.8% of the respondents believe that they can solve their problems by their self.

Table 39

Table Revealing the Belief of the Respondents on being Perplexed by their Contradictory Thoughts

Response	Frequency	Percent
Always	230	63.9
Most of Times	120	33.3
Never	10	2.8
Total	360	100

The above shown table indicates that 63.9% of the respondents believe that they are being perplexed by their contradictory thoughts always, 33.3% of the respondents believe that they are being perplexed by their contradictory thoughts most of times and 2.8%of the respondents believe that they are never being perplexed by their contradictory thoughts.

Table 40

Table Exhibiting the Opinion of the Respondents on not able to Continue any Task for Long

Response	Frequency	Percent
Always	310	86.1
Most of Times	20	5.6
Sometimes	30	8.3
Total	360	100

The above shown table indicates that 86.1% of the respondents believe that they are not able to continue any task for long always, 8.3% of the respondents believe that they are not able to continue any task for long sometimes and 5.6% of the respondents believe that they are not able to continue any task for long most of times.

Table 41

Table Presenting the Feeling of being Secured Admist of Friends or Groups by the Respondents

Response	Frequency	Percent
Most of Times	10	2.8
Sometimes	40	11.1
Never	310	86.1
Total	360	100

The above shown table indicates that 86.1% of the respondents feel that they are never felt secured admist of friends or groups,11.1% of the respondents feel that they are feeling secured admist of friends or groups sometimes and 2.8% of the respondents feel that they are feeling secured admist of friends or groups most of times.

Discussion

Gibson and Jefferson (2006) Studied and find out that adolescence self - concept is supported by the influence of peers, mentors, family and involvement community. This result is contrary to the present study.

Table 42

Table Demonstrating the Opinion of the Respondents on the Feeling that they not become Hopeless even When They Fail

Response	Frequency	Percent
Always	20	5.6
Most of Times	10	2.8
Sometimes	10	2.8
Never	320	88.9
Total	360	100

The above table indicates that 88.9 % of the respondents feel that they never become hopeless when they fail, but 5.6 % of the respondents feel that they do not become hopeless even when they fail always, 2.8% of the respondents feel that they do not become hopeless even when they fail most of times and 2.8% of the respondents feel that they do not become hopeless even when they fail sometimes.

Table 43

Table Indicating the Opinion of the Respondents on not Getting Influenced even by Reasonable Arguments

Response	Frequency	Percent
Always	310	86.1
Most of Times	40	11.1
Never	10	2.8
Total	360	100

The above table indicates that 86.1 % of the respondents feel that they are not getting influenced even by reasonable arguments always, 11.1% of the respondents feel that they are not getting influenced even by reasonable arguments most of times and 2.8% of the respondents feel that they get influenced even by reasonable arguments.

Table 44

Table Revealing the Feeling of the Respondents on being Afraid of Imaginary Calamities

Response	Frequency	Percent
Always	330	91.7
Most of Times	10	2.8
Sometimes	20	5.6
Total	360	100

The above table indicates that 91.7% of the respondents feel that they are afraid of imaginary calamities always,5.6% of the respondents feel that they are afraid of imaginary calamities sometimes and 2.8% of the respondents feel that they are afraid of imaginary calamities most of times.

Table 45

Table Exhibiting the Feeling of the Respondents on whether World is a Good Place for Living

Response	Frequency	Percent
Most of Times	30	8.3
Sometimes	100	27.8
Never	230	63.9
Total	360	100

The above table indicates that 63.9% of the respondents feel that world is not a good place for living, 27.8% of the respondents feel that world is a good place for living sometimes and 8.3% of the respondents feel that world is a good place for living most of times.

Table 46

Table Depicting the Respondents' Feeling on being Fully Enthusiastic on Thinking about Achieving Self Objectives

Response	Frequency	Percent
Most of Times	10	2.8
Sometimes	20	5.6
Never	330	91.7
Total	360	100

The above table indicates that 91.7% of the respondents does not feel fully enthusiastic on thinking about achieving self objectives, 5.6% of the respondents feel fully enthusiastic on thinking about achieving self objectives sometimes and 2.8% of the respondents feel fully enthusiastic on thinking about achieving self objectives most of times.

Table 47

Table Showing the Feeling of Respondents on do not Getting Disappointed with Common Worries of Daily Life

Response	Frequency	Percent
Always	10	2.8
Most of Times	20	5.6
Sometimes	140	38.9
Never	190	52.8
Total	360	100

The above table shows that 52.8% of the respondents feel that they get disappointed with common worries of daily life, but 38.9% of the respondents opine that they do not get disappointed with common worries of daily life sometimes, 5.6% of the respondents opine that they do not get disappointed with common worries of daily life most of times and 2.8% of the respondents opine that they do not get disappointed with common worries of daily life always.

Table 48

Table Demonstrating the Feeling of Respondents on their Mood Changes

Response	Frequency	Percent
Always	330	91.7
Most of Times	20	5.6
Never	10	2.8
Total	360	100

The above table shows that 91.7% of the respondents feel that their mood changes momentarily always, 5.6% of the respondents feel that their mood changes momentarily most of times and 2.8% of the respondents opine that their mood never changes momentarily.

Table 49

Table Presenting the Feeling of Respondents that their Intimacy with their Group Community is Increasing

Response	Frequency	Percent
Most of Times	110	30.6
Sometimes	20	5.6
Never	230	63.9
Total	360	100

The above table shows that 63.9% of the respondents feel that their intimacy with their group community is not increasing, but 30.6% of the respondents feel that their intimacy with their group community is increasing most of times and 5.6% of the respondents feel that their intimacy with their group community is increasing sometimes.

Table 50

Table Indicating the Opinion of Respondents on Feeling Pleasure in Taking Responsibilities

Response	Frequency	Percent
Always	10	2.8
Never	350	97.2
Total	360	100

The above table shows that 97.2% of the respondents feel that they never feel pleasure in taking responsibilities and 2.8% of the respondents feel that they feel pleasure in taking responsibilities always.

Table 51

Correlation Table for the Mental Health and Home Environment of the Adolescent Girls

		TOT Part 1	TOT2
totpart1	Pearson Correlation	1	.348**
	Sig. (2-tailed)		.000
	N	360	360
TOT2	Pearson Correlation	.348**	1
	Sig. (2-tailed)	.000	
	N	360	360

**. Correlation is significant at the 0.01 level (2-tailed).

Correlation is positive

The table indicates that the mental health of the respondents is positively correlated to the home environment of the adolescents, which means the home environment affects and plays a key role in the mental health of the adolescent girls. The correlation test applied shows that there is a positive correlation as the correlation is significant at the 0.01 level (2-tailed).

Discussion

Deb et al. (2015) have conducted study and their research revealed that parental traits were found to be negatively influenced by mental health. This result is contradictory to the findings of the present study.

Table 52

Correlation Table Presenting the Home Environment and Personality Traits of the Adolescent Girls

		TOT2	ATOT
TOT2	Pearson Correlation	1	-.545**
	Sig. (2-tailed)		.000
	N	360	360
ATOT	Pearson Correlation	-.545**	1
	Sig. (2-tailed)	.000	
	N	360	360

**. Correlation is significant at the 0.01 level (2-tailed).

Correlation is negative

The above stated table shows that there is negative correlation which means home environment of the respondents is not influenced and related to the personality traits of the adolescents. The correlation is significant at the 0.01 level (2-tailed).

Table 53

Correlation Table Depicting the Personality Traits and Mental Health of the Respondents

		A TOT	TOT Part1
ATOT	Pearson Correlation	1	-.413**
	Sig. (2-tailed)		.000
	N	360	360
totpart1	Pearson Correlation	-.413**	1
	Sig. (2-tailed)	.000	
	N	360	360

**. Correlation is significant at the 0.01 level (2-tailed).

Correlation is negative

The table indicates that there is negative correlation between personality traits and mental health of the respondents which means mental health is not related to and influenced by personality traits of the adolescents.

Discussion

For-Wey Lung (2006) conducted a study to examine the personality traits and mental health among Taiwanese military students with adjustment disorder. Among 641 students, differences between students was found with adjustment disorder and those without adjustment disorder were statistically significant in terms of their premorbid personality and mental health. Different kinds of school discipline appear to be a precipitating factor for adjustment disorder; however, neurotic, introvert, and psychotic traits appear to be predisposing factors for adjustment disorder. This results says that personality traits are positively correlated to mental health, but it is contradictory to the results of the present study.

Table 54

Chi Square test Showing home Environment and Mental Health of the Respondents

			Home environment			Total
			Good	Normal	Poor	
Mental health	High	Count	20	30	0	50
		Expected Count	6.9	34.7	8.3	50.0
	Normal	Count	30	140	40	210
		Expected Count	29.2	145.8	35.0	210.0
	Low	Count	0	80	20	100
		Expected Count	13.9	69.4	16.7	100.0
Total		Count	50	250	60	360
		Expected Count	50.0	250.0	60.0	360.0

Chi-Square Tests

	Value	Df	Asymp. Sig. (2-sided)
Pearson Chi-Square	50.651[a]	4	.000
Likelihood Ratio	64.416	4	.000
Linear-by-Linear Association	34.097	1	.000
N of Valid Cases	360		

a. 0 cells (0.0%) have expected count less than 5. The minimum expected count is 6.94.

Symmetric Measures					
		Value	**Asymp. Std. Error[a]**	**Approx. T[b]**	**Approx. Sig.**
Nominal by Nominal	Phi	.375			.000
	Cramer's V	.265			.000
Interval by Interval	Pearson's R	.308	.040	6.129	.000[c]
Ordinal by Ordinal	Spearman Correlation	.297	.041	5.883	.000[c]
N of Valid Cases		360			

a. Not assuming the null hypothesis.

b. Using the asymptotic standard error assuming the null hypothesis.

c. Based on normal approximation.

There is association between home environment and mental health of students.

Pearson chi-square value is 50.651. It means that home environment is closely associated to mental health of the adolescents.

Table 55

Chi Square test Demonstrating Personality traits and Mental Health of Adolescent Girls

			Personality traits		Total
			Low	High	
Mental health	High	Count	20	30	50
		Expected Count	16.7	33.3	50.0
	Normal	Count	90	120	210
		Expected Count	70.0	140.0	210.0
	Low	Count	10	90	100
		Expected Count	33.3	66.7	100.0
Total		Count	120	240	360
		Expected Count	120.0	240.0	360.0

Chi-Square Tests			
	Value	**Df**	**Asymp. Sig. (2-sided)**
Pearson Chi-Square	34.071[a]	2	.000
Likelihood Ratio	39.151	2	.000
Linear-by-Linear Association	22.307	1	.000
N of Valid Cases	360		
a. 0 cells (0.0%) have expected count less than 5. The minimum expected count is 16.67.			

There is an association between personality traits and mental health of the adolescent girls and the chi square value is 34.071

Symmetric Measures

		Value	Asymp. Std. Error[a]	Approx. T[b]	Approx. Sig.
Nominal by Nominal	Phi	.308			.000
	Cramer's V	.308			.000
Interval by Interval	Pearson's R	.249	.046	4.870	.000[c]
Ordinal by Ordinal	Spearman Correlation	.260	.045	5.104	.000[c]
N of Valid Cases		360			

a. Not assuming the null hypothesis.

b. Using the asymptotic standard error assuming the null hypothesis.

c. Based on normal approximation.

Table 56

T-Test Presenting Mental Health and Psychotism

	PA mean	N	Mean	Std. Deviation	Std. F
	Low	180	90.9444	11.89090	
	High	180	88.2222	4.11504	

	Levene's Test for Equality of Variances		t-test for Equality of Means					
	F	Sig.	t	df	Sig. (2-tailed)	Mean Difference	Std. Error Difference	95% Inte D Lower
qual variances ssumed	77.665	.000	2.903	358	.004	2.72222	.93787	.87780
qual variances ot assumed			2.903	221.269	.004	2.72222	.93787	.87393

be noted from the mean table that the Mental health is good for the children who have lower psych
he F value 77.665 is significant at 0.01 level.

Table 57

T-Test Exhibiting Mental Health and Depression

Depression	N	Mean	Std. Deviation	Std. Err
Low	250	90.0800	10.33542	.65
High	110	88.4545	4.50002	.42

	Levene's Test for Equality of Variances		t-test for Equality of Means					
	F	Sig.	t	df	Sig. (2-tailed)	Mean Difference	Std. Error Difference	95% Int D Lowe
ual variances umed	23.108	.000	1.584	358	.114	1.62545	1.02632	-.392
ual variances not umed			2.079	357.981	.038	1.62545	.78191	.087

noted from the mean table that the Mental Health is better for the children who have lower Depression F value 23.108 is significant at 0.01 level.

Table 58

T- Test Representing Mental Health and Extroversion

Extroversion	N	Mean	Std. Deviation	Std. Er
Low	240	87.5833	3.84769	.2
High	120	93.5833	13.77770	1.2

	Levene's Test for Equality of Variances		t-test for Equality of Means					
	F	Sig.	t	df	Sig. (2-tailed)	Mean Difference	Std. Error Difference	95% In
								Low
qual variances ssumed	293.874	.000	-6.282	358	.000	-6.00000	.95513	-7.878
qual variances not ssumed			-4.680	128.365	.000	-6.00000	1.28201	-8.536

e noted from the mean table that the Mental Health is better for the children who have Higher Extrover
e F value 293.874 is significant at 0.01 level and

Table 59

T -Test Indicating Mental Health and Emotional Instability

Emotional Instability	N	Mean	Std. Deviation	Std. Er
Low	260	90.4615	10.25629	.6
High	100	87.3000	3.24271	.3

	Levene's Test for Equality of Variances		t-test for Equality of Means					
	F	Sig.	t	df	Sig. (2-tailed)	Mean Difference	Std. Error Difference	95% Int D
								Low
ıual variances sumed	45.059	.000	3.023	358	.003	3.16154	1.04594	1.10
ıual variances not sumed			4.428	349.382	.000	3.16154	.71396	1.75

noted from the mean table that the Mental Health is better for the children who have Lower Emotiona
icant as the F value 45.059 is significant at 0.01 level.

Table 60

T- Test Showing Mental Health and Social Desirability

Social Desirability	N	Mean	Std. Deviation	Std. E
Low	250	88.5200	6.27432	.3
High	110	92.0000	12.95015	1.

	Levene's Test for Equality of Variances		t-test for Equality of Means					
	F	Sig.	t	df	Sig. (2-tailed)	Mean Difference	Std. Error Difference	95% Inte D Lower
ual variances sumed	68.296	.000	-3.434	358	.001	-3.48000	1.01335	-5.4728
ual variances t assumed			-2.683	132.062	.008	-3.48000	1.29695	-6.0454

ed)	Mean Difference	Std. Error Difference	95% Confidence Interval of the D	
			Lower	Up
	-3.48000	1.01335	-5.47287	-1.48
	-3.48000	1.29695	-6.04548	-.91

e noted from the mean table that the Mental Health is better for the children who have Higher Soc
ficant as the F value 68.296 is significant at 0.01 level.

Table 61

Chi-Square Test Presenting Medium of Instruction and Total Members in Family

			Total Members in Family			Total
			3	4	5	
Medium	Malayalam	Count	80	80	0	160
		Expected Count	84.4	71.1	4.4	160.0
	English	Count	110	80	10	200
		Expected Count	105.6	88.9	5.6	200.0
Total		Count	190	160	10	360
		Expected Count	190.0	160.0	10.0	360.0

Chi-Square Tests	Value	df	Asymp. Sig. (2-sided)
Pearson Chi-Square	10.421[a]	2	.005
Likelihood Ratio	14.166	2	.001
Linear-by-Linear Association	.000	1	1.000
N of Valid Cases	360		

a. 1 cells (16.7%) have expected count less than 5. The minimum expected count is 4.44.

Symmetric Measures		Value	Approx. Sig.
Nominal by Nominal	Phi	.170	.005
	Cramer's V	.170	.005
N of Valid Cases		360	

There is a small impact of medium of instruction and members in family. There is significant association between medium of instruction and members in family. Chi square value is 10.421 which is significant.

Table 62

Chi-Square Test Displaying Medium of Instruction and Father's Education

			Father's Education			Total
			Primary	Secondary	Higher Secondary	
Medium	Malayalam	Count	40	110	10	160
		Expected Count	26.7	115.6	17.8	160.0
	English	Count	20	150	30	200
		Expected Count	33.3	144.4	22.2	200.0
Total		Count	60	260	40	360
		Expected Count	60.0	260.0	40.0	360.0

Chi-Square Tests	Value	df	Asymp. Sig. (2-sided)
Pearson Chi-Square	18.606[a]	2	.000
Likelihood Ratio	18.986	2	.000
Linear-by-Linear Association	18.202	1	.000
N of Valid Cases	360		

a. 0 cells (0.0%) have expected count less than 5. The minimum expected count is 17.78.

Symmetric Measures		Value	Approx. Sig.
Nominal by Nominal	Phi	.227	.000
	Cramer's V	.227	.000
N of Valid Cases		360	

The above table shows that there is a significant association between father's education and medium of instruction and the value is 18.606 and the impact correlation coefficient is 0.227.

Table 63

Chi-Square Test Exhibiting Medium of Instruction and Mother's Education

			Mother's Education				Total
			Primary	Secondary	Higher Secondary	Graduate and above	
Medium	Malayalam	Count	70	90	0	0	160
		Expected Count	40.0	84.4	31.1	4.4	160.0
	English	Count	20	100	70	10	200
		Expected Count	50.0	105.6	38.9	5.6	200.0
Total		Count	90	190	70	10	360
		Expected Count	90.0	190.0	70.0	10.0	360.0

Chi-Square Tests	Value	df	Asymp. Sig. (2-sided)
Pearson Chi-Square	105.158[a]	3	.000
Likelihood Ratio	136.396	3	.000
Linear-by-Linear Association	98.949	1	.000
N of Valid Cases	360		

a. 1 cells (12.5%) have expected count less than 5. The minimum expected count is 4.44.

Symmetric Measures		Value	Approx. Sig.
Nominal by Nominal	Phi	.540	.000
	Cramer's V	.540	.000
N of Valid Cases		360	

It is clear from the above table that there is a significant association between medium of instruction and mother's education. The chi square value is 105.158 and the influence phi cramer's V is 0.540

Table 64

Anova Test for Medium of Instruction and Home Environment

	Sum of Squares	df	Mean Square	F	Sig.
Between Groups	3.556	1	3.556	.027	.870
Within Groups	47312.000	358	132.156		
Total	47315.556	359			

The above table shows that there is no significant difference in the opinion on home environment of students based on their medium of instruction as the p value is > 0.05.

Table 65

Anova Test Exhibiting Home Environment and Age

	Sum of Squares	df	Mean Square	F	Sig.
Between Groups	2774.972	2	1387.486	11.121	.000
Within Groups	44540.583	357	124.764		
Total	47315.556	359			

Age	Mean	N	Std. Deviation
15	91.0000	20	13.33772
16	81.4583	240	10.15355
17	78.3000	100	12.91816
Total	81.1111	360	11.48034

The above table shows that there is a significant difference in the opinion of students on home environment based on their age as the F value 11.121. The mean table shows that the more the age the opinion decreases, as it is significant at 0.01.

Table 66

Anova Test Showing Home environment and Birth Order

	Sum of Squares	df	Mean Square	F	Sig.
Between Groups	2336.870	3	778.957	6.165	.000
Within Groups	44978.686	356	126.345		
Total	47315.556	359			

Birth Order	Mean	N	Std. Deviation
First	82.3846	130	9.32230
Second	78.5833	120	14.66407
Third	84.3750	80	8.97165
Fourth	77.0000	30	7.92203
Total	81.1111	360	11.48034

The above table shows that there is a significant difference in the opinion of students on home environment based on their birth order as the F value 6.165 is significant at 0.01. The mean table shows that the student of third birth order have better opinion and the second is first child and it is further low for the second child and fourth child.

Table 67

Anova Test Presenting Home Environment and Father's Education

	Sum of Squares	df	Mean Square	F	Sig.
Between Groups	9711.709	2	4855.855	46.100	.000
Within Groups	37603.846	357	105.333		
Total	47315.556	359			

Father's Education	Mean	N	Std. Deviation
Primary	77.0000	60	11.28971
Secondary	79.8462	260	10.55851
Higher Secondary	95.5000	40	5.57007
Total	81.1111	360	11.48034

It is clear from the table shows that there is a significant difference in the opinion of students on home environment based on father's education, the F value 46.100 is significant at 0.01 level.

The mean table shows that the more the father's education, better the home environment.

Table 68

Anova Test Displaying Home Environment and Mother's Education

	Sum of Squares	df	Mean Square	F	Sig.
Between Groups	5501.955	3	1833.985	15.615	.000
Within Groups	41813.601	356	117.454		
Total	47315.556	359			

Mother's Education	Mean	N	Std. Deviation
Primary	81.2222	90	10.92135
Secondary	79.9474	190	10.83046
Higher Secondary	80.8571	70	11.43892
Graduate and above	104.0000	10	.00000
Total	81.1111	360	11.48034

It is clear from the table shows that there is a significant difference in the opinion of students on home environment based on mother's education, the F value 15.615 is significant at 0.01 level.

The mean table shows that if the mother is educated the home environment is better.

Table 69

Anova Test Demonstrating Home Environment and Family Monthly Income

	Sum of Squares	df	Mean Square	F	Sig.
Between Groups	17136.181	3	5712.060	67.380	.000
Within Groups	30179.375	356	84.774		
Total	47315.556	359			

Family Monthly Income	Mean	N	Std. Deviation
25000 to 50000	95.0000	30	7.09541
10000 to 25000	92.0000	40	2.77350
5000 to 10000	74.0000	130	11.79278
Below 5000	81.5625	160	8.11838
Total	81.1111	360	11.48034

It is clear from the table shows that there is a significant difference in the opinion of students on home environment based on mother's education, the F value 67.380 is significant at 0.01 level.

The mean table shows that if the monthly family income is more there is a better home environment.

Table 70

Anova Test Exhibiting Home Environment and Number of Family Members

	Sum of Squares	df	Mean Square	F	Sig.
Between Groups	300.161	2	150.080	1.140	.321
Within Groups	47015.395	357	131.696		
Total	47315.556	359			

The above table shows that there is no significant difference in the opinion on home environment of students based on the number of members at home as the p value is > 0.05.

Table 71

Factor Analysis for Home Environment

Factor Analysis was done for pinion on Home Environment with 22 Items Following Field's (2005) Guidelines to Reduce the Number of Variables.

KMO and Bartlett's Test

Kaiser-Meyer-Olkin Measure of Sampling Adequacy.		.391
Bartlett's Test of Sphericity	Approx. Chi-Square	4920.262
	Df	231
	Sig.	.000

The results of factor analysis of opinion on home environment of the respondents shows that KMO test confirm 39% of the sample adequacy, Bartlett's test of spharcity was also significant. So it can be concluded that the data was suitable for the Factor Analysis.

Total Variance Explained

Component	Extraction Sums of Squared Loadings			Rotation Sums of Squared Loadings		
	Total	% of Variance	Cumulative %	Total	% of Variance	Cumulative %
1	4.688	21.311	21.311	3.758	17.084	17.084
2	2.750	12.500	33.811	2.602	11.828	28.911
3	2.284	10.384	44.195	2.395	10.886	39.797
4	1.903	8.650	52.845	2.295	10.431	50.228
5	1.676	7.617	60.462	2.252	10.234	60.462

Extraction Method: Principal Component Analysis

From above table it can be seen that 5 factors or subscales had been extracted initially. Each factor had Eigen Values greater than one. Factor 1 accounted for the most variance among all factors (21.31%), followed by the variance in the second factor (which accounted for 12.5%), followed by the variance in the third factor (which accounted for

10.38%), followed by the variance in the fourth factor (which accounted for 8.65%) and variance in the fifth factor (which accounted for 7.61%). Together, the 5 factors accounted for 60.46% of the variability of the 22 items. After rotation loadings, the percentage of total variance accounted for was 60.46%.

It is visible in the above table that, the Rotated Component Matrix Table displays 5 factors and 22 items of Home environmental scale. Items with loadings greater than 0.5 were included in the table. According to Isaac and Michael (1990), to have a meaningful factor, at least three items should load on it. In this research, 1 factors loaded with 7 items, 1 factor loaded with 4 items and rest 3 factors loaded with 3 items each.

Factor 1 :- Parents's influence

Factor 2:- Criticism / communication

Factor 3:- difference of opinions / disagreements

Factor 4:- absence of equality among siblings

Factor 5:- Lack of freedom/problem to express feelings

Component Transformation Matrix

Component	1	2	3	4	5
1	.794	.403	.124	.386	.207
2	-.124	.577	-.591	.130	-.534
3	-.475	.354	.650	.462	-.115
4	.353	-.126	.420	-.321	-.761
5	-.059	.603	.189	-.720	.281

Extraction Method: Principal Component Analysis.

Rotation Method: Varimax with Kaiser Normalization

The present study resulted that parent's influence is the important factor in home environment, followed by it comes communication factor at home. The other factors are to difference of opinion, absence of equality among siblings and lack of freedom factor accounted respectively and less loaded factor is lack of freedom.

Discussion

Leug and Shek (2012) have done study and found that parenting style, parental control, family functioning and parental sacrifice for children's education were positively related to adolescent psychosocial competence. This result is same as the result of the present study.

Table 72

Comparison Table Showing Mental health Scores based on the Personality Dimension- Psychotism and Home Environment of the Respondents

Home Environment			Psychotism				Total	
			Low	%	High	%		%
Good	Mental health	High	10	5.55	0	0	10	2.77
		Normal	20	11.11	20	11.11	40	11.11
	Total		30	16.66	20	11.11	50	13.88
Normal	Mental health	High	20	11.11	0	0	20	5.55
		Normal	110	61.11	120	6.66	230	63.88
	Total		130	72.22	120	66.66	250	69.44
Poor	Mental health	Normal	20	11.11	40	22.22	60	16.66
	Total		20	11.11	40	22.22	60	16.66
Total	Mental health	High	30	16.66	0	0	30	8.33
		Normal	150	83.33	180	100	330	91.66
	Total		180		180		360	100

When Home Environment is good, mental health of respondents ranged from high to normal.

At high mental health, the personality dimension Psychotism is low at 5.55%. When mental health is normal it is low at 11.11% and high at 11.11%.

When home environment is normal, Mental Health of respondents ranged from high to normal and when mental health is high, the personality dimension Psychotism is low at 11.11%. When mental health is in normal stage, then Psychotism is low at 61.11% and high at 6.66%. When home environment is poor, Mental health of respondents is normal and Psychotism is low at 11.11% and high at 22.22%.

Table 73

Comparison Table for Mental Health Scores Based on the Personality Dimension-Depression and Home Environment of the Respondents

Home Environment			Depression				Total	
			Low	**%**	**High**	**%**		**%**
Good	Mental health	High	10	4	0	0	10	2.77
		Normal	10	4	30	27.27	40	11.11
	Total		20	8	30	27.27	50	13.88
Normal	Mental health	High	20	8	0	0	20	5.55
		Normal	160	64	70	63.63	230	63.88
	Total		180	72	70	63.63	250	69.44
Poor	Mental health	Normal	50	20	10	9.09	60	16.66
	Total		50	20	10	9.09	60	16.66
Total	Mental health	High	30	12	0	0	30	8.33
		Normal	220	88	110	100	330	91.66
	Total		250	100	110	100	360	100

When Home Environment is good, mental health of respondents ranged from high to normal, at high Mental health, the personality dimension depression is low at 4.0%. When Mental health is normal it is low at 4.0% and high at 27.27%.

When home environment is normal, Mental Health of respondents ranged from high to normal and when mental health is high, the personality dimension depression is low at 8.0%. When mental health is in normal stage, then depression is low at 64.0% and high at 63.63%.

When home environment is poor, mental health of respondents is normal and depression is low at 20.0% and high at 9.09%.

Table 74

Comparison table Indicating Mental Health Scores based on the Personality Dimension Extroversion and Home Environment of the Respondents

<table>
<tr><th colspan="3" rowspan="2">Home Environment</th><th colspan="4">Extroversion</th><th>Total</th><th></th></tr>
<tr><th>Low</th><th>%</th><th>High</th><th>%</th><th></th><th>%</th></tr>
<tr><td rowspan="3">Good</td><td rowspan="2">Mental health</td><td>High</td><td>0</td><td>0</td><td>10</td><td>8.33</td><td>10</td><td>2.77</td></tr>
<tr><td>Normal</td><td>30</td><td>12.5</td><td>10</td><td>8.33</td><td>40</td><td>11.11</td></tr>
<tr><td colspan="2">Total</td><td>30</td><td>12.5</td><td>20</td><td>16.66</td><td>50</td><td>13.88</td></tr>
<tr><td rowspan="3">Normal</td><td rowspan="2">Mental health</td><td>High</td><td>0</td><td>0</td><td>20</td><td>16.66</td><td>20</td><td>5.55</td></tr>
<tr><td>Normal</td><td>150</td><td>62.5</td><td>80</td><td>66.66</td><td>230</td><td>63.88</td></tr>
<tr><td colspan="2">Total</td><td>150</td><td>62.5</td><td>100</td><td>83.33</td><td>250</td><td>69.44</td></tr>
<tr><td rowspan="2">Poor</td><td>Mental health</td><td>Normal</td><td>60</td><td>25</td><td>0</td><td>0</td><td>60</td><td>16.66</td></tr>
<tr><td colspan="2">Total</td><td>60</td><td>25</td><td>0</td><td>0</td><td>60</td><td>16.66</td></tr>
<tr><td rowspan="2">Total</td><td rowspan="2">Mental health</td><td>High</td><td>0</td><td>0</td><td>30</td><td>25</td><td>30</td><td>8.33</td></tr>
<tr><td>Normal</td><td>240</td><td>100</td><td>90</td><td>75</td><td>330</td><td>91.66</td></tr>
<tr><td></td><td colspan="2">Total</td><td>240</td><td>100</td><td>120</td><td>100</td><td>360</td><td>100</td></tr>
</table>

When Home Environment is good, mental health of respondents ranged from high to normal, at high Mental health, the personality dimension extroversion is high at 8.33% and when Mental health is normal it is low at 12.5% and high at 8.33%. When home environment is normal, Mental Health of respondents ranged from high to normal and when mental health is high, the personality dimension extroversion is high at 16.66%.When mental health is in normal stage, then extroversion is low at 62.5% and high at 66.66%. When home environment is poor, mental health of respondents is normal and extroversion is low at 25.0%.

Discussion

Sangeeta (2006) studied the relationship between introversion - extroversion and mental health on 600 boys studying in tenth standard in high and higher secondary school of Jammu city. The results indicate that extroversion tendencies enhance the mental health whereas introversion tendencies deteriorate mental health. These results were found similar to the inferences of the present research study.

Table 75

Comparison table for Mental Health Scores Based on the Personality Dimension - Emotional Instability and Home Environment of the Respondents

Home Environment			Emotional Instability				Total	
			Low	%	High	%		
Good	Mental health	High	10	3.84	0	0	10	2.77
		Normal	40	15.38	0	0	40	11.11
	Total		50	19.23	0	0	50	13.88
Normal	Mental health	High	20	7.69	0	0	20	5.55
		Normal	150	57.69	80	80	230	63.88
	Total		170	65.38	80	80	250	69.44
Poor	Mental health	Normal	40	15.38	20	20	60	16.66
	Total		40	15.38	20	20	60	16.66
Total	Mental health	High	30	11.53	0	0	30	8.33
		Normal	230	88.46	100	100	330	91.66
	Total		260	100	100	100	360	100

When Home Environment is good, mental health of respondents ranged from high to normal, at high mental health, the personality dimension emotional instability is low at 3.84%. When mental health is normal it is low at 15.38%.

When home environment is normal, Mental Health of respondents ranged from high to normal and when mental health is high, the personality dimension emotional instability is low at 7.69%. When mental health is in normal stage, then emotional instability is low at 57.69% and high at 80.00%.

When home environment is poor, mental health of respondents is normal and emotional instability is low at 15.38% and high at 20%.

Table 76

Comparison table for Mental Health Scores Based on the Personality Dimension-Social Desirability and Home Environment of the Respondents

Home Environment			Social Desirability				Total	%
			Low	%	High	%		
Good	Mental health	High	10	4	0	0	10	2.77
		Normal	20	8	20	18.18	40	11.11
	Total		30	12	20	18.18	50	13.88
Normal	Mental health	High	0	0	20	18.18	20	5.55
		Normal	170	68	60	54.54	230	63.88
	Total		170	68	80	72.72	250	69.44
Poor	Mental health	Normal	50	20	10	9.09	60	16.66
	Total		50	20	10	9.09	60	16.66
Total	Mental health	High	10	4	20	18.18	30	8.33
		Normal	240	96	90	81.81	330	91.66
	Total		250	100	110	100	360	100

When Home Environment is good, mental health of respondents ranged from high to normal, at high mental health, the personality dimension social desirability is low at 4%. When mental health is normal it is low at 8% and high at 18.18%.

When home environment is normal, Mental Health of respondents ranged from high to normal and when mental health is high, the personality dimension social desirability is high at 18.18%. When mental health is in normal stage, then social desirability is low at 68.00% and high at 54.54%.

When home environment is poor, mental health of respondents is normal and social desirability is low at 20% and high at 9.09%.

CHAPTER V

FINDINGS, IMPLICATIONS AND CONCLUSIONS

Introduction

There are certain complex set of reasons, most of what is known about adolescent girls focuses on the problems they face. The fact that many adolescent girls are showing remarkable strength, resiliency, and hardness during the stressful time of adolescence needs to be explored. Instead of focusing on the storm and stress of adolescence, a new understanding of adolescent girls that affirms their strength and resilience needs to be developed. Although the current day risks and stresses in the lives of adolescent girls must be understood, they should not be the defining factors in discussions of adolescent girls. There must be a focus on what is working for adolescent girls, and why to assist adolescent girls in navigating these risks during their development.

Results Related to Hypotheses

1. There is no significant difference in the Mental Health and Home Environment of the adolescent girls.

   Chi square test was applied to test the hypothesis. The results reveals that there is an association between home environment and mental health of the adolescent girls and the chi square value is 23.71.

   Hence the null hypothesis is rejected.

2. There is no significant difference in the Home environment and mental health of students.

   Chi square test was applied to check the hypothesis. Results shows that there is an association between personality traits and mental health of the adolescent girls and the chi square value is 34.071.

   Hence the null hypothesis is rejected.

3. There is no significant difference in the personality traits and mental health of the adolescent girls.

One Way Annova test was applied to check the hypothesis. Results shows that there is a significant difference in the mental health based on father's education. F= 61.140 is significant at 0.05 level. The mean value is high when father's education is more. Hence student's mental health increased when father's education is good.

Hence the null hypothesis is rejected

4. There is no significant difference in the educational qualification of the father and mental health of their wards.

   One Way Annova test was applied to check the hypothesis. Results indicate that there is a significant difference in the mental health based on father's education. F= 61.140 is significant at 0.05 level. The mean value is high when father's education is more. Hence student's mental health inventory increased when father's education is good.

   Hence the null hypothesis is rejected.

5. There is a no significant difference in the mental health of students based on their age.

   One Way Anova test was applied to check the hypothesis. Results shows that there is a significant difference on the mental health of students based on their age as the significant value (of F = 3.298) 0.038 < 0.05.The mean value of the mental health inventory shows that students at the age of 15 have more mental health and the second highest is 16 years old children and it is comparatively low for the students at the age of 17.

   Hence the null hypothesis is rejected.

6. There is no significant difference in the mental health of students based on their birth order.

   One Way Anova test was applied to check the hypothesis It is clear that there is no significant difference in the mental health of students based on their birth order as the significance value is > 0.05.

   Hence the null hypothesis is rejected.

7. There is no significant difference in the mental health of students based on the monthly family income.

One Way Anova test was administered to check the hypothesis. There is a significant difference in the mental health of students based on the monthly family income, as the sig level (of F =11.014) is < 0.01.The mean value shows that the mental health is more when the income of the Family increases.

Hence the null hypothesis is rejected.

8. There is no significant difference in the opinion of students on home environment based on their age.

   One Way Anova test was applied to check the hypothesis. There is a significant difference in the opinion of students on home environment based on their age as the F value 11.121 is significant at 0.01. The mean table shows that the more the age the opinion decreases.

   Hence the null hypothesis is rejected.

9. There is no significant difference in the opinion of students on home environment based on father's education.

   One Way Anova test was carried out to check the hypothesis. There is a significant difference in the opinion of students on home environment based on father's the more the father's education, better the home environment.

   Hence the null hypothesis is rejected.

10. There is no significant difference in the opinion on home environment of students based on the number of members at home.

    One Way Anova test was administered to check the hypothesis. The test results shows that there is no significant difference in the opinion on home environment of students based on the number of members at home as the p value is > 0.05.

    Hence the null hypothesis is accepted.

Findings of the Study

Findings Related to Personal Details

- Majority of the respondents 66.7% belong to the age group of 16 years.
- Majority of the respondents 55.6% have been from Malayalam medium of instruction.
- Majority of the respondents 33.1 % are first born in birth order.
- Majority of the respondents fathers 72.2% are secondary educated.
- Majority of the respondents mothers 52.8 % are secondary educated.

Findings Related Mental Health Status

- Vast majority 94% of them feel lack of confidence always.
- Vast majority 88.9% of them get excited very easily most of the times.
- Vast majority 88.9% of them believe that they are not able to take quick decision on any subject always.
- Vast majority 91.7% of the respondents feel that situations are continuously going against them always.
- Vast majority 91.7% of the respondents feel that they never have affection and attachment with their neighbors.
- Majority 63.9 % of the respondents opine that they never make adjustments according to the circumstances,
- Majority 69.4 % of the respondents feel that they are losing self-respect sometimes.
- Majority 63.9 % of the respondents feel that they keep worrying about trivial matters for long time sometimes.
- Vast majority 97.2% of the respondents feel hesitation in meeting others always.
- Majority 41.7% of the respondents feel that they are not able to fully utilize their ability in performing duties sometimes,

- Majority 69.4% of the respondents feel that even in adverse circumstances, they act without keeping in view of the real facts most of the times.
- Vast majority 91.7% of the respondents feel that they get irritated always.
- Vast majority 91.7% of the respondents opine that they feel insecure always.
- Vast majority 91.7% of the respondents feel that they are much worried about their responsibilities always.
- Vast majority 94.4% of the respondents opine that they feel depressed or dejected always.
- Majority72.2% of the respondents feel that they are able to utilize their reasoning even in difficult times most of the times.
- Majority 66.7% of the respondents feel that their relations with others are not satisfactory most of the times.
- Vast majority 88.9% of the respondents feel inferiority complex always.
- Results reveal that 100.0% of the respondents opined that they feel to be lost in the world of imagination always.
- Vast majority 80.6% of the respondents are anxious about their future sometimes.
- Vast majority 66.7% of the respondents opine that they are never enraged by the slightest unfavourable task.
- Majority 69.4 % of the respondents believe that their confidence never varies high in quantity.
- Majority 55.6% of the respondents are willing to fight the problems of life most of times.
- Analysis of data reveals that 72.2% of the respondents believe that they can solve their problems by their self most of times.
- Results of analysis shows that 63.9% of the respondents believe that they are being perplexed by their contradictory thoughts always.

- Vast majority 86.1% of the respondents believe that they are not able to continue any task for long always.
- Vast majority 86.1% of the respondents feel that they are never felt secured admist of friends or groups.
- Vast majority 88.9 % of the respondents feel that they never become hopeless when they fail.
- Vast majority 86.1 % of the respondents feel that they are not getting influenced even by reasonable arguments always.
- Vast majority 91.7% of the respondents feel that they are afraid of imaginary calamities always.
- Vast majority 63.9% of the respondents feel that world is not a good place for living.
- Vast majority 91.7% of the respondents does not feel fully enthusiastic on thinking about achieving self objectives.
- Vast majority 91.7% of the respondents does not feel fully enthusiastic on thinking about achieving self objectives.
- Majority 52.8% of the respondents feel that they get disappointed with common worries of daily life.
- Vast majority 91.7% of the respondents feel that their mood changes momentarily always.
- Majority 63.9% of the respondents feel that their intimacy with their group community is not increasing.
- Vast majority 97.2% of the respondents feel that they never feel pleasure in taking responsibilities.

Findings Related to T-test

- The T- test is significant as the F value 77.665 is significant at 0.01 level and it is to be noted from the mean table that the Mental health is good for the children who have lower Psychotism.
- The T- test is significant as the F value 23.108 is significant at 0.01 level and it is to be noted from the mean table that the Mental Health is better for the children who have lower Depression.
- The T -test is significant as the F value 293.874 is significant at 0.01 level and it is to be noted from the mean table that the Mental Health is better for the children who have Higher Extroversion.
- The T-test is significant as the F value 45.059 is significant at 0.01 level and it is to be noted from the mean table that the Mental Health is better for the children who have Lower Emotional Instability.
- The T-test is significant as the F value 68.296 is significant at 0.01 level and it is to be noted from the mean table that the Mental Health is better for the children who have Higher Social Desirability.

Findings Related To Chi-Square

- Chi square test applied shows that there is association between Home environment and mental health of students. Pearson chi-square value is 50.651.
- Chi square test applied shows that there is an association between personality traits and mental health of the adolescent girls and the chi square value is 34.071.
- There is significant association between medium of instruction and members in family.
- Chi square value is 10.421 which is significant.
- There is a significant association between father's education and medium of instruction and the value is 18.606 and the impact correlation coefficient is 0.227.
- It is clear from the above table that there is a significant association between medium of instruction and mother's education. The chi square value is 105.158 and the influence phi cramer's V is 0.540

- Findings of the One Way Anova test applied show that there is a significant difference on the mental health of students based on their age as the significant value (of $F = 3.298$) $0.038 < 0.05$.

- The One Way Anova test applied shows that the mental health of adolescent girls is more when there are 4 members and it is low when this increases. i.e., students from family of two children father and mother feel better compared to family with grandparents or other relatives and it is also low with students of single child family.

- It is evident from the One Way Anova test of the mental health that students at the age of 15 have more mental health and the second highest is 16 years old children and it is comparatively low for the students at the age of 17.

- There is no significant difference in the opinion on home environment of students based on their medium of instruction as the p value is > 0.05.

- There is a significant difference in the opinion of students on home environment based on their age as the F value 11.121 is significant at 0.01. The mean table shows that the more the age the opinion decreases.

- There is a significant difference in the opinion of students on home environment based on their birth order as the F value 6.165 is significant at 0.01. The mean table shows that the student of third birth order have better opinion and the second is first child and it is further low for the second child and fourth child.

- There is a significant difference in the opinion of students on home environment based on father's education, the F value 46.100 is significant at 0.01 level. The mean table shows that the more the father's education, better the home environment.

- There is a significant difference in the opinion of students on home environment based on mother's education, the F value 15.615 is significant at 0.01 level.

- The mean table shows that if the mother is educated the home environment is better.

- There is a significant difference in the opinion of students on home environment based on mother's education, the F value 67.380 is significant at 0.01 level.

- The mean table shows that if the monthly family income is more there is a better home environment.
- The above table shows that there is no significant difference in the opinion on home environment of students based on the number of members at home as the p value is > 0.05.
- Factor analysis was done on the home environment factors of adolescent girls. Factor 1 that is **parent's influence** accounted for the most variance among all factors (21.31%), followed by the variance in the second factor that is **difference of opinion** which accounted for 12.5%). Together, the 5 factors accounted for 60.46% of the variability of the 22 items. After rotation loadings, the percentage of total variance accounted for was 60.46%. According to Isaac and Michael (1990), to have a meaningful factor, at least three items should load on it. In this research, factor 1 – parent's influence: loaded with 7 items, factor 3: difference of opinion loaded with 4 items and rest of the 3 factors like Absence of equality among siblings, Lack of freedom/problem to express feelings, Criticism / communication loaded with 3 items each.

The factors are:

Factor 1:- Parents's influence

Factor 2:- Criticism / communication

Factor 3:- difference of opinions / disagreements

Factor 4:- absence of equality among siblings

Factor 5:- Lack of freedom/problem to express feelings

The Pearson correlation test done between the Home Environment and Personality traits of the adolescent girls shows that the Correlation is negative. Correlation is significant at the 0.01 level.

The Pearson correlation test between the Mental Health and Home Environment of the adolescent girls clearly states that the Correlation is positive. Correlation is significant at the 0.01 level.

Figure 9

Figure Showing Changes in Adolescent Girls

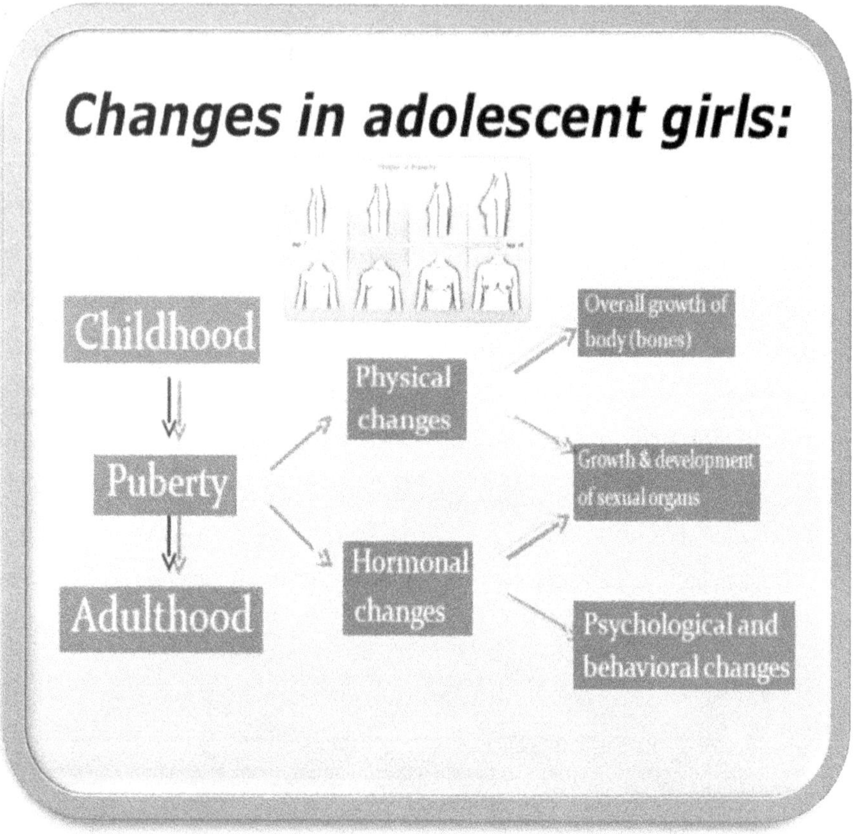

Summary of the Study

Adolescence is a developmental transition between childhood and adulthood. It is generally considered to begin at about age ten and to end in the late teens. There are two most important factors for studying adolescents. This is the period of growth spurt where maximum changes can be observed in an individual as compared to the other phases of life the first factor in understanding and studying adolescents is the rapid changes that occur during this period and the influence that have on the growth and development of adolescents. This stage of life is called critical period and also as the stage of growth spurt. Adolescence is also an emotional and social process and so it is said, adolescence begins in biology and ends in culture.The storm and stress often associated with the teenage years have been called adolescent rebellion that may encompass not only conflict within the family but a general alienation from adult society and hostility towards the values. Since adolescence is a crucial period for emotional life, because frontal lobes, which are important for regulating limbic impulse, mature during this period and since it's the time of exploration (of their own bodies, of one's capabilities and potential) and experimentation in sexual relationship's alcohol and tobacco use. It is extremely important to understand emotional and intelligence aspect in adolescents. Understanding the various factors affecting overall development of adolescents is as important as understanding the significance of studying adolescents. Taking this view into consideration studying psychosocial problems of adolescent girls from the social work perspective.

Adolescent girls receive contradictory expectations from different aspects of their life parents, teacher, peers, the media, and themselves. They are to be sexy and fashionable but at the same time remain good girls. They are to find off aggressive female attention while simultaneously meeting teacher's expectations of non-aggressive behavior. Females are to put domestic life first at the same time that they prepare for financial independence. Girls struggle with these conflicting messages, trying to figure out whom to please in their everyday live. While many girls, especially those of lower socio-economic status, have adult responsibilities such as cleaning, cooking, and caring for younger children, they are discouraged from speaking up at school and claiming this same type of authority.

Discussions of the Results

The researcher had adopted questionnaire method for the purpose of collecting data from the respondents. It was used to find out the mental health of adolescent girls in relation to their home environment and personality traits. The questionnaire consists of 4 parts:

- First part consists of **personal profile.**
- The second part consists of **Mental Health Inventory** which consists of questions relating to mental health dimensions and it is 55 questions together. The Mental health inventory was constructed by Jagdish & Srivastav, in 1983. It was utilized to access positive aspects of mental health. Each items from 1 to 56 given in the test booklet to be rated on 4 point rating scale. It covers the following 6 dimensions of sound mental health. They are Positive Self-Evaluation, Perception of Reality, Integration of Personality, Autonomy, Group Oriented Attitudes and Environment Mastery.
- The third part consists of **Personality Inventory** that was constructed and standardized by B.L. Dubey, P. Dwivedi and S. K. Verma in 1988 and was used in this study. The Inventory consists of 50 statements. The purpose of the inventory is to measure the dimensions of personality like extroversion, psychotism, emotional instability, depression and social desirability.
- The fourth part consists of **Home Environment Inventory** for understanding the perceptions of adolescents regarding various areas of home environments. It was constructed by Dr. Ms. Sarla Java. It is 5 point scale with 74 items and was modified by the researcher herself. The modified inventory consists of 22 items together about the aspects of the home environment correlates.

Results states there is a significant Correlation between home environment and mental health of the adolescent girls. Home Environment positively correlated to mental health, it means that mental health influenced by the home environment condition of the adolescents.

Correlation test done between the Home Environment and Personality traits of the adolescent girls shows that the Correlation is negative. It is evident that there is no significant relationship between Home Environment and Personality Traits of the Adolescent.

Parent's influence and difference of opinion are the most important factors in determining the home environment. Parents play key role in the life of adolescents and the most loaded and important factor according to analysis was parent's influence and the least loaded factor was lack of freedom factor.

Results reveal that if the monthly family income is more there is a better home environment.

Tests exhibits that if the mother is educated the home environment is better.

The mean table shows that the more the father's education, better the home environment.

Results shows that the student of third birth order have better opinion about matters, ordinal position is important in determining personality and mental health of the Adolescents.

It was found, mean table shows that the more the age the opinion decreases.

It is evident from the One Way Anova test of the mental health that students at the age of 15 have more mental health.

The mental health of adolescent girls is more when there are 4 members and it is low when this increases. i.e., students from family of two children father and mother feel better compared to family with grandparents or other relatives and it is also low with students of single child family.

There is a significant difference on the mental health of students based on their age.

There is an association between personality traits and mental health of the adolescent girls

There is an association between home environment and mental health of the adolescent girls and the chi square value.

Mental health is good for the children who have lower Psychotism.

Mental Health is better for the children who have lower Depression.

Mental Health is better for the children who have Higher Extroversion.

Mental Health is better for the children who have Lower Emotional Instability.

Mental Health is better for the children who have Higher Social Desirability.

Social Work Intervention

Social work is a professional and academic discipline that seeks to improve the quality of life and well-being of an individual, group or community by intervening through research, policy, crisis intervention, community organizing, direct practice, and teaching on behalf of those afflicted with poverty or any real or perceived social injustices and violations of their civil liberties and human rights. Research is often focused on areas such as human development, social policy, public administration, psychotherapy, counseling, program evaluation, and international and community development. Social workers are organized into local, national, continental and international professional bodies. Social work, an interdisciplinary field includes theories from economics, education, sociology, law, medicine, philosophy, politics, anthropology and psychology.

The social work profession promotes social change, problem - solving in human relationships and empowerment and liberation of people to enhance well-being. Utilizing theories of human behavior and social systems, social work intervenes at the points where people interact with their environments. Principles of human rights and social justice are fundamental to social work. Social work in its various forms addresses the multiple, complex transaction between people and their environment. Its mission is to enable all people to develop their full potential, enriching their lives and prevent dysfunction. Professional social work is focused on problem solving and change. Social work is an interrelated system of values, theory and practice. Social work grew out of humanitarian and democratic ideals, and its values are based on respect for the equality worth, and dignity of all people. In Modern society all men and women, young and old, adolescent and matured, sick and handicapped, are facing challenges in their lives and struggling hard with them to adjust. Social work is, a help rendered to any person or group, who or which is suffering from any disability, mental, physical, emotional or moral, so that the individual or group so helped is enable to help himself or herself.

Figure 10

Figure Representing Social Work at a Glance

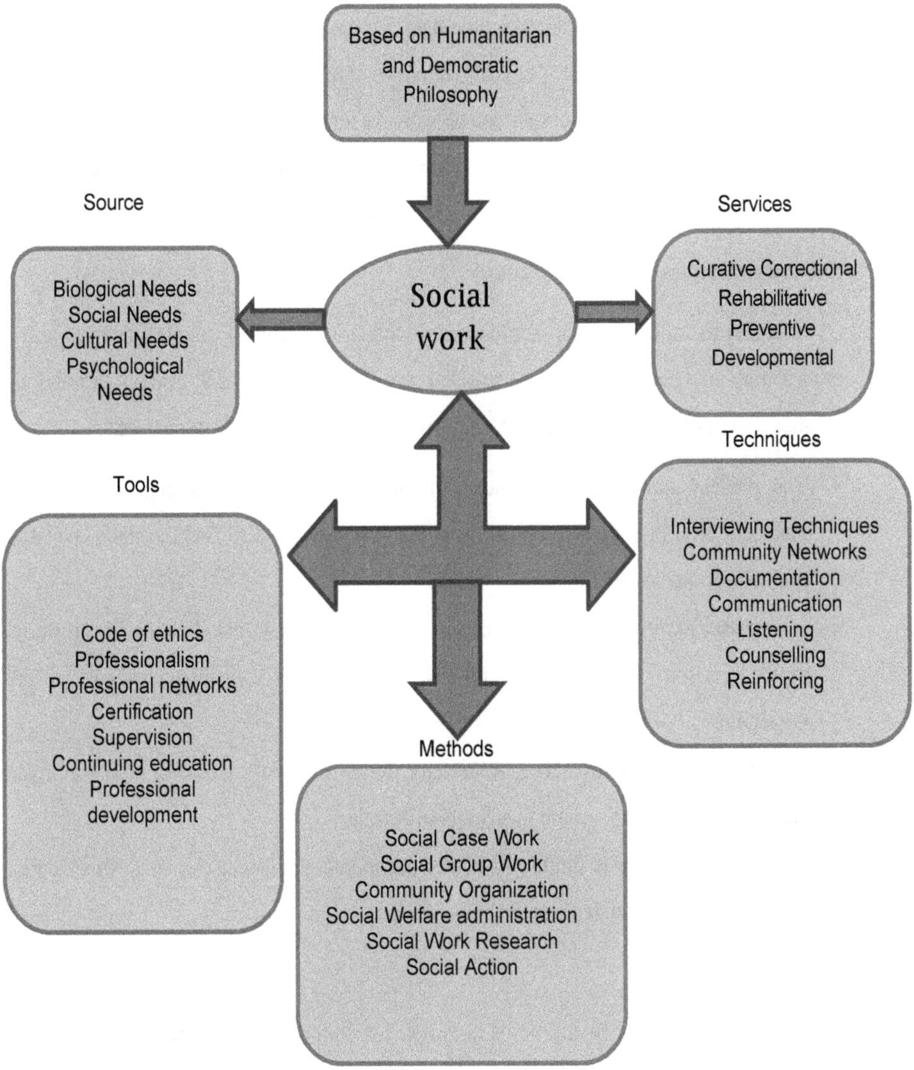

Social work interventions range from primarily person-focused psychosocial processes for involvement in social policy, planning and development. These include counselling, clinical social work, group work, social pedagogical work, and family treatment and therapy as well as efforts to help people obtain services and resources in the community. Interventions also include agency administration, community organization and engaging in social and political action to impact social policy and economic development. The holistic focus of social work is universal, but the priorities of social work practice will vary from country to country and from time to time depending on cultural, historical, legal and socio-economic conditions.

Recommendations for further Studies

Indepth study on the adolescence with low level of mental health, home environment and personality can be selected separately as samples to find out the reasons for their low level of mental health, home environment, personality dimensions.

- The present study was confirmed only to girls of higher secondary schools of Palakkad city. Studies may be conducted among boys also to find out their level and problem of mental health.
- A comparative study among all schools of the district can also be carried out throw more light on mental health and relation to socio - economic status of the respondents.
- As it was a micro study school s and city limits were only included it can be made vast by conducting this same in schools of Kerala.
- The present study was limited to higher secondary schools it can be further carried out among college students also.

Suggestions

Adolescence can be a time of high risk for children, where new found freedoms can result in decisions that drastically open up or close off life opportunities. Parental issues at this stage of parenting include dealing with "rebellious" teenagers, who didn't know freedom while they were smaller. In order to prevent all these, it is important to build a trusting relationship with them. This can be achieved by planning and spending fun activities together, keeping promises, do not nag at him or her about their past mistakes and try to listen and talk to them, no matter how busy you are. When a trusting relationship is built, they are more likely to approach parent for help when faced with negative peer pressure. Also, try to built a strong foundation to help child to resist negative peer pressure, it is important to build up their self-esteem: praise child's strength instead of focusing on their weakness acknowledge child's efforts, do not simply focus on the final result when they notice that then they will turn to their peers for acceptance and comfort. There are not enough mental health professionals trained to work specifically with children, adolescents, and their families:

- Support education and training of more mental health professionals with the skills to deal effectively with the mental health needs of children, adolescents, and their families.
- Support workforce training on the advanced tools and methods that have been found to be safe and most effective for diagnosis and treatment of mental health problems in children and adolescents. Training should emphasize sensitivity to family needs, cultural differences, and what is appropriate for children at different ages.
- Support training of front line providers, including those in schools, child care settings, primary health care settings, juvenile justice system, and child protective services, to screen for and recognize mental health problems in youth and to take appropriate action.
- Support training for researchers and encourage interdisciplinary research that will find new behavioral, pharmacological, and multiple component treatment approaches to child and adolescent mental health problems.
- Adolescents must be trained in physical exercises to improve mental health. **Stuart and Mavis (2011)** states that mall but consistent associations between sedentary life style and poorer mental health.

Managing Adolescent Mental Health Issues

Enhancing social skills, problem-solving skills and self-confidence can help prevent mental health problems such as conduct disorders, anxiety, depression and eating disorders as well as other risk behaviors including those that relate to sexual behavior, substance abuse, and violent behavior. Health workers need to have the competencies to relate to young people, to detect mental health problems early, and to provide treatments which include counseling, cognitive-behavioral therapy and, where appropriate, psychotropic medication.

Treatment

Activity therapies

Activity therapies, also called recreation therapy and occupational therapy, promote healing through active engagement. Making crafts can be a part of occupational therapy. Walks can be a part of recreation therapy.

Bio-feedback

Biofeedback is a process of gaining control of physical processes and brainwaves. It can be used to decrease anxiety, increase well-being, increase relaxation, and other methods of mind-over-body control.

Expressive therapies

Expressive therapies are a form of psychotherapy that involves the arts or art-making. These therapies include music therapy, art therapy, dance therapy, drama therapy, and poetry therapy.

Group therapy

Group therapy involves any type of therapy that takes place in a setting involving multiple people. It can include psychodynamic groups, activity groups for expressive therapy, support groups (including the twelve-step program), problem-solving and psycho education groups.

Psychotherapy

Psychotherapy is the general term for scientific based treatment of mental health issues based on modern medicine. It includes a number of schools, such as gestalt therapy, psychoanalysis, cognitive behavioral therapy and dialectical behavioral therapy.

Meditation

The practice of mindfulness meditation has several mental health benefits, such as bringing about reductions in depression, anxiety and stress. Mindfulness meditation may also be effective in treating substance use disorders. Further, mindfulness meditation appears to bring about favorable structural changes in the brain.

Spiritual counseling

Spiritual counselors meet with people in need to offer comfort and support and to help them gain a better understanding of their issues and develop a problem-solving relation with spirituality. These types of counselors deliver care based on spiritual, psychological and theological principles.

Stress Relief Activities

Adolescents must be taught stress relief activities. This could help them to maintain balance by themselves.

Figure 11

Figure Exhibiting Stress Relief Activities

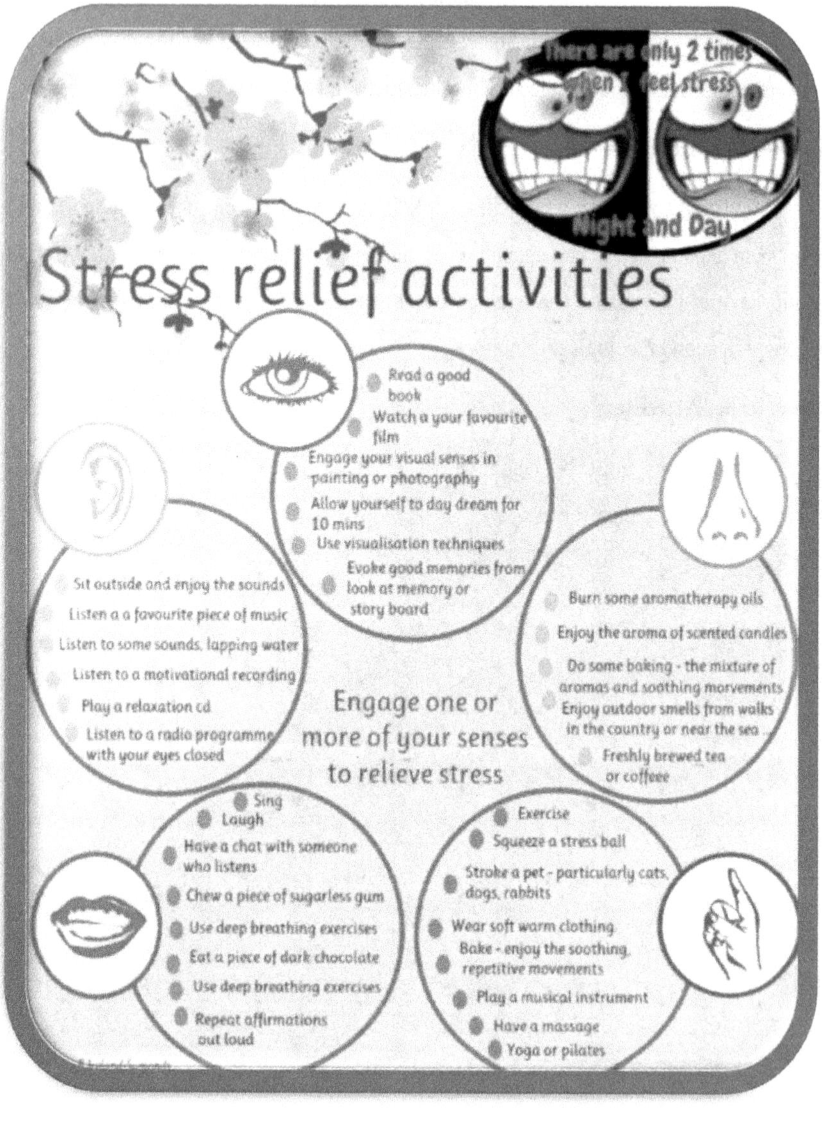

Conclusion

A discussion of the problems of adolescence should be useful for various reasons. In the first place, it may be helpful to adolescents themselves. The intelligent youth who is actually in the midst of the adjustments here considered may profit from the definite, impersonal formulation of the persistent problems of youth everywhere. Too often the struggles of an adolescent are made harder by the idea that he or she alone is being called upon to pass through these experiences. To realize that these are universal problems about which generalizations may be offered is in itself helpful.

CPSIA information can be obtained
at www.ICGtesting.com
Printed in the USA
LVHW051639200423
744807LV00010B/387

9 787815 206865